SCIENTIFIC AMERICAN EXPLORES BIG IDEAS

Understanding Pandemics and Epidemics

The Editors of *Scientific American*

SCIENTIFIC AMERICAN EDUCATIONAL PUBLISHING

New York

Published in 2024 by Scientific American Educational Publishing
in association with **The Rosen Publishing Group**
2544 Clinton Street, Buffalo, NY 14224

Contains material from Scientific American®, a division of Springer Nature America, Inc., reprinted by permission, as well as original material from The Rosen Publishing Group®.

First Edition

Scientific American
Lisa Pallatroni: Project Editor

Rosen Publishing
David Kuchta: Compiling Editor
Michael Moy: Senior Graphic Designer

Cataloging-in-Publication Data
Names: Scientific American Editors (New York, New York), editor.
Title: Understanding pandemics and epidemics / the editors of Scientific American.
Description: First edition. | New York : Scientific American Educational Publishing, 2024. | Series: Scientific American explores big ideas | Includes bibliographical references and index. | Audience: Grades 10-12
Identifiers: LCCN 2023034883 | ISBN 9781725350311 (library binding) | ISBN 9781725350304 (paperback) | ISBN 9781725350328 (ebook)
Subjects: LCSH: Epidemics–Juvenile literature. | Pandemics–Juvenile literature. | COVID-19 Pandemic, 2020–Juvenile literature. | Public health–Juvenile literature. | Communicable diseases–Juvenile literature.
Classification: LCC RA653.5 .U53 2024 | DDC 614.4/973–dc23/eng/20230824
LC record available at https://lccn.loc.gov/2023034883

Manufactured in the United States of America
Websites listed were live at the time of publication.

Cover: Prostock-studio/Shutterstock.com

CPSIA Compliance Information: Batch # CWSA24.
For Further Information contact Rosen Publishing at 1-800-237-9932.

CONTENTS

Introduction 6

Section 1: Lessons From the Past 7

1.1 100 Years after the Lethal 1918 Flu Pandemic, We Are Still Vulnerable 8
By Catharine I. Paules and Anthony S. Fauci

1.2 The 1918 Flu Faded in Our Collective Memory: We Might 'Forget' the Coronavirus, Too 12
By Scott Hershberger

1.3 Lessons from Past Outbreaks Could Help Fight the Coronavirus Pandemic 19
By Sara Goudarzi

1.4 Stories from a Past Pandemic 24
By The Editors

1.5 Millions of People Living with HIV Are Alive, Thanks to a 20-Year Public Health Effort 30
By Lauren J. Young

1.6 HIV Care Has Improved Dramatically—But Not for Everyone 37
By David Malebranche

1.7 Lessons from AIDS for the COVID-19 Pandemic 41
By William A. Haseltine

Section 2: The Science and Medicine of COVID-19 52

2.1 How China's 'Bat Woman' Hunted Down Viruses from SARS to the New Coronavirus 53
By Jane Qiu

2.2 A High-Speed Scientific Hive Mind Emerged from the COVID Pandemic 63
By Joseph Bak-Coleman and Carl T. Bergstrom

2.3 An mRNA Pioneer Discusses How Her Work Led to the COVID Vaccines 67
By Tanya Lewis

2.4 Messenger RNA Therapies Are Finally Fulfilling Their Promise 72
By Drew Weissman

2.5 Pandemic-Era Research Will Pay Off for Years 75
By Britt Glaunsinger

2.6 COVID Revealed the Fragility of American Public Health 76
By Wendy E. Parmet

2.7 COVID Pushed Global Health Institutions to Their Limits 78
By Lawrence O. Gostin

Section 3: How COVID-19 Changed Society 84

3.1 COVID Has Made Global Inequality Much Worse 85
By Joseph E. Stiglitz

3.2 COVID Has Created a Perfect Storm for Fringe Science 88
By David Robert Grimes

3.3 COVID Changed the World of Work Forever 92
By Christina Maslach and Michael P. Leiter

3.4 How a Virus Exposed the Myth of Rugged Individualism 94
By Robin G. Nelson

3.5 How the Pandemic Remade Science Journalism 98
By Tanya Lewis

3.6 Introducing 21 Ways COVID Changed the World 102
By Jen Schwartz

Section 4: Meanwhile, Other Epidemics 105

4.1 The Biggest Health Problem: Obesity 106
By Mercedes Carnethon

4.2 The Opioid Epidemic Is Surging among Black People because of Unequal Access to Treatment 109
By Melba Newsome and Gioncarlo Valentine

4.3 Doctors Need to Learn to Talk about Suicide 118
By Rodolfo Bonnin and Leonard M. Gralnik

4.4 Why Does Ebola Keep Showing Up in the Democratic Republic of the Congo? 122
By Dina Fine Maron

4.5 Ebola Outbreak in Uganda Surges, but the Country Has a Plan 126
By Paul Adepoju

4.6 "Their Lives Are Worth More Than Ours": Experts in Africa Slam Global Response to Monkeypox 131
By Paul Adepoju

4.7 We Can't Let Monkeypox Turn into a Repeat of COVID 136
By Muhammad Jawad Noon

Section 5: What Lies Ahead 140

5.1 Tick- and Mosquito-Borne Diseases Are Increasing Dramatically 141
By Kacey C. Ernst

5.2 Want to Prevent Another Coronavirus Epidemic? 146
By William A. Haseltine

5.3 The Next Zika 149
By Marta Zaraska

5.4 COVID Is Here to Stay 153
By Christine Crudo Blackburn

Glossary 155

Further Information 156

Citations 157

Index 158

INTRODUCTION

In 2017, Dr. Anthony Fauci coauthored an article for *Scientific American*, reproduced in this volume, warning about "the inevitable pandemic viruses that will emerge in the future." At the time, Dr. Fauci was widely known and well-regarded in medical circles, but he was not the household name that he would become three years later. In 2017 there was no questioning of his integrity in the U.S. Senate, no #FireFauci, no threats to his life.

Epidemics and pandemics do that to communities: they widen the fault lines in a society and bring underlying tensions to the fore. During the Black Death, simmering antisemitism boiled over into massacres. Epidemics and pandemics also bring social change. Waves of cholera in the 19th century spurred the rise of indoor plumbing and clean drinking water. And pandemics sometimes cause the fall of entire societies. Old World diseases devastated indigenous peoples and made European conquest of the Americas possible.

This book focuses heavily on the COVID-19 pandemic, but it also looks both backward and forward. Section 1 examines historical precedents in order to make comparisons with the COVID-19 pandemic. Section 2 focuses on the strengths and weaknesses of the healthcare system as it confronted the COVID-19 crisis. Section 3 shows how COVID-19 revealed and widened the fissures in our society. Section 4 looks at other, ongoing epidemics that threaten our health, while Section 5 examines what potential epidemics and even pandemics may lie ahead. As Dr. Fauci warned, we are still, and always will be, vulnerable.

Healthcare and medicine never exist in a vacuum. They are influenced by the scientific questions we ask and those we fail to ask, by the choices we make in taking some medical threats seriously and overlooking others. Never has that been more true than during the COVID-19 pandemic. Our own experiences and the lessons we've learned may help us better respond to "the inevitable pandemic viruses that will emerge in the future."

Section 1: Lessons From the Past

1.1 100 Years after the Lethal 1918 Flu Pandemic, We Are Still Vulnerable
By Catharine I. Paules and Anthony S. Fauci

1.2 The 1918 Flu Faded in Our Collective Memory: We Might 'Forget' the Coronavirus, Too
By Scott Hershberger

1.3 Lessons from Past Outbreaks Could Help Fight the Coronavirus Pandemic
By Sara Goudarzi

1.4 Stories from a Past Pandemic
By The Editors

1.5 Millions of People Living with HIV Are Alive, Thanks to a 20-Year Public Health Effort
By Lauren J. Young

1.6 HIV Care Has Improved Dramatically—But Not for Everyone
By David Malebranche

1.7 Lessons from AIDS for the COVID-19 Pandemic
By William A. Haseltine

100 Years after the Lethal 1918 Flu Pandemic, We Are Still Vulnerable

By Catharine I. Paules and Anthony S. Fauci

In 2018 the world will mark the 100th anniversary of the most devastating infectious disease event in recorded history: the 1918 influenza pandemic.

The severity of the event, which caused an estimated 50 million to 100 million deaths worldwide, likely resulted from several factors: First, most of the global population probably had no preexisting immune protection to the brand-new virus that had emerged. Evidence from the study of viral genes suggests the 1918 flu virus originated from an avian source and then somehow adapted to circulate efficiently in humans. Second, inherent properties of this virus may have contributed to its pathogenicity—the mechanisms by which it caused illness. Finally, efforts to control the spread of the pandemic and prevent morbidity and mortality were limited by conditions and technologies of the time. Crowding and poor sanitation allowed for rampant disease transmission, especially in areas where access to health care was limited. Antivirals to treat influenza were not available in 1918, and infections often were complicated by fatal bacterial pneumonias for which there were no effective antibiotics.

Further, protective vaccines—the cornerstone of modern influenza prevention—were still decades in the future. And even though we now have such vaccines, they likely would not be effective against a 1918-like virus. One hundred years later, we must reexamine our approach to influenza vaccines so we can avert a repeat of that worldwide catastrophe.

Over the past 100 years, apart from vaccines, substantial advances have been made in public health and health care infrastructure, particularly intensive care capacity. In addition, we now have antiviral drugs for influenza, antibiotics for secondary bacterial infections and influenza vaccines. Despite these developments, however, seasonal influenza epidemics still cause some 12,000 to 56,000 deaths each year in the U.S. These seasonal influenza viruses continually evolve by accumulating mutations in the genes that code for surface proteins and/or swapping genes with other influenza viruses. When the result is a small or modest change in the virus, it is referred to as an antigenic drift. We attempt to mitigate the burden of influenza by developing new seasonal vaccines for both hemispheres each year that target the influenza viruses surveillance suggests will be most common in the upcoming influenza season. Even though these vaccines are updated frequently, they may be only 40 to 60 percent effective against seasonal influenza viruses. And in some years vaccine–virus mismatches occur because new variants appear and spread in the interval between vaccine formulation and deployment. In these cases, vaccine effectiveness is considerably lower.

Importantly, seasonal influenza vaccines may provide little or no protection against pandemic influenza viruses where the new virus is considerably different from circulating seasonal viruses. Pandemic viruses typically arise from a process referred to as an antigenic shift, in which the new virus acquires, usually from animal influenza viruses, one or more genes that are entirely novel (as seems to have happened in 1918, when all eight pandemic virus genes were novel).

After 1918 three influenza pandemics associated with antigenic shifts occurred: in 1957, 1968 and 2009. In each of these instances, however, the new viruses emerged via the mixing or reassortment of animal influenza virus genes with those of the 1918-descended viruses already circulating in the human population. Likely explanations for the lesser severity of the last three pandemics compared with that of 1918 include lower viral pathogenicity, partial preexisting immunity to the new viruses and improvements in public health infrastructure and medical treatment. Vaccines were not a major factor, as effective vaccines were not available until well after the peak of each pandemic. The three recent influenza pandemics remind us that new pandemics are inevitable, and that current seasonal vaccines are unlikely to prevent or significantly control them.

We also must address the issue of "pre-pandemic" influenza viruses, that is, those that threaten to emerge to cause pandemics but that have not (yet) done so. In this regard, human infections with avian influenza viruses, such as Asian lineage A(H5N1) and A(H7N9), have occurred with increasing frequency over the past two decades. The risk of human adaptation of these viruses to cause a future pandemic remains unknown but vigilance is called for. Pre-pandemic vaccines against various strains of H5N1 and H7N9 viruses have been developed and in some cases stockpiled; similar to seasonal influenza viruses, however, these avian strains are subject to antigenic drift within their avian hosts. For example, many of the H7N9 avian viruses that have jumped species from poultry to cause human infections in China in 2017 have changed significantly from 2013 avian strains. As a result, the human immune responses elicited by a vaccine developed against the 2013 A(H7N9) virus may not be effective against its 2017 strains.

The remarkable capacity of influenza viruses to undergo antigenic drift or shift to overcome and escape human population immunity leaves us vulnerable to a public health disaster potentially as serious as the 1918 pandemic. To meet this global health challenge, scientists are working to develop "universal influenza vaccines"—new types of inoculations that can provide protection not only against changing seasonal influenza viruses but also against the inevitable pandemic viruses that will emerge in the future.

Recently the National Institute of Allergy and Infectious Diseases (NIAID) at the U.S. National Institutes of Health convened a scientific agenda-setting workshop with leading experts in the influenza field to address the need for better influenza vaccines. Among many hurdles to developing a universal vaccine, the most formidable is our incomplete understanding of the immune responses that protect people against influenza, including the role of immunity at mucosal surfaces.

Current influenza vaccines generate an immune response focused disproportionately on viral surface proteins called hemagglutinins. This response is mediated by antibodies, Y-shaped proteins made by the immune system to neutralize pathogens. Each influenza virus has one of the 18 different known hemagglutinin subtypes, and an antibody response to a vaccine or natural infection is specific to that subtype, leaving individuals vulnerable to attack by viruses containing hemagglutinins against which they have previously not been vaccinated for or infected by. Also, influenza virus hemagglutinins can mutate over time so that previously made antibodies no longer recognize them.

One approach to a universal influenza vaccine under active consideration is to design them to generate antibody responses to parts of the virus that are common to all influenza virus strains and do not readily change by mutation. One such component of influenza that remains relatively constant from virus to virus is a specific region of the hemagglutinin protein called the stalk, or stem. It is also important to clarify how other parts of the immune system such as immune cells work together with antibodies to protect against influenza. Although hurdles in the development of such universal vaccines are daunting, we are optimistic that we can apply existing tools and experimental approaches to meet the challenge.

As we approach the centennial of the 1918 influenza pandemic, let us be reminded of the importance of this line of research in preventing a repeat of one of the most disastrous events in the history of global health.

The views expressed are those of the author(s) and are not necessarily those of Scientific American.

About the Authors

Catharine I. Paules is a medical officer in the Office of the Director at the National Institute of Allergy and Infectious Diseases.

Anthony S. Fauci is director of the National Institute of Allergy and Infectious Diseases.

The 1918 Flu Faded in Our Collective Memory: We Might 'Forget' the Coronavirus, Too

By Scott Hershberger

In 1924 Encyclopædia Britannica published a two-volume history of the 20th century thus far. More than 80 authors—professors and politicians, soldiers and scientists—contributed chapters to *These Eventful Years: The Twentieth Century in the Making as Told by Many of Its Makers*. But the book's sprawling 1,300 pages never mention the catastrophic influenza pandemic that had killed between 50 million and 100 million people worldwide only five years earlier. And many history textbooks in subsequent decades just note the 1918–1919 flu pandemic as an aside when discussing World War I, if at all.

Until quite recently, the pandemic had remained strangely faint in the public sphere, compared with other momentous events of the 20th century. Monuments and federal holidays commemorate people lost in both World Wars. Many popular museums and blockbuster movies recount the sinking of the *Titanic* and the Apollo moon missions. But the same cannot be said for the 1918 flu (often referred to as the "Spanish flu" because of mistaken beliefs about its origin). Of course, the pandemic was not forgotten entirely: many today are aware it occurred or even know of ancestors who succumbed to it. But the event seems to form a disproportionately small part of our society's narrative of its past.

That such a devastating pandemic could become so dormant in our collective memory puzzled Guy Beiner, a historian at Ben-Gurion University of the Negev in Israel, prompting him to spend decades researching its legacy. "We have an illusion. We believe that if an event is historically significant—if it affects many, many people, if it changes the fate of countries in the world, if many people die from it—then it will inevitably be remembered," he says.

"That's not at all how it works. And the Spanish flu is exactly a warning for that."

Beiner began collecting books about the 1918 pandemic 20 years ago. For a long time, they emerged in a very slow trickle. But now, as the world reckons with COVID-19, he can hardly keep up with the outpouring of both nonfiction and fiction. "I have, in my office, three stacks [of novels] waiting for me–huge stacks," he says. Previously a niche topic even among historians, the 1918 flu has been compared to the current pandemic in terms of the fatality rate, apparent effectiveness of masks and social distancing, and potential economic impact. In March 2020 alone, the English-language Wikipedia page for "Spanish flu" garnered more than 8.2 million views, shattering the pre-2020 monthly record of 144,000 views during the pandemic's 2018 centennial.

The worldwide "forgetting" and ongoing rediscovery of the 1918 flu provide a window into the science of collective memory. And they offer tantalizing clues about how future generations might regard the current coronavirus pandemic.

What is Collective Memory?

Pioneered in the early 20th century by sociologist Maurice Halbwachs, the study of collective memory has garnered widespread interest across the social sciences in recent years. Henry Roediger III, a psychologist at Washington University in St. Louis, defines collective memory as "how we remember ourselves as part of a group ... that forms our identity." Groups such as nations, political parties, religious communities and sports fandoms, he explains, weave events from their collective past into a narrative that reinforces individual members' shared sense of who they are.

Researchers often use open-recall methods to study groups' collective memory of well-known historical events. For example, Roediger and his colleague James Wertsch, also at Washington University in St. Louis, asked Americans and Russians to name the 10 most important events of World War II. Americans most often cited the attack on Pearl Harbor, the atomic bombings of Japan and the Holocaust. Most Russians highlighted the Battle of Stalingrad, the Battle of Kursk and the Siege of Leningrad. The only event that appeared on both lists was D-Day, known in Russia as "the opening of the second front." The events most strongly recalled by people in each country, the researchers say, reflect that nation's narrative framework, or schema, for remembering the past.

Such a study could indicate what specifics about the 1918 flu people are aware of. But "as far as I know, nobody's done it," Wertsch says. "If you did a survey, you would come up with nothing." Even in making comparisons with COVID-19, he says, few individuals can cite significant details about the earlier pandemic. Wertsch notes that collective memory seems to depend largely on narratives with a clear beginning, middle and end. "If there's one cognitive instrument that is the most ubiquitous, most natural..., it's narrative," he says. "Not all human cultures have arithmetic number systems, let alone calculus. But all human cultures use narratives."

For the countries engaged in World War I, the global conflict provided a clear narrative arc, replete with heroes and villains, victories and defeats. From this standpoint, an invisible enemy such as the 1918 flu made little narrative sense. It had no clear origin, killed otherwise healthy people in multiple waves and slinked away without being understood. Scientists at the time did not even know that a virus, not a bacterium, caused the flu. "The doctors had shame," Beiner says. "It was a huge failure of modern medicine." Without a narrative schema to anchor it, the pandemic all but vanished from public discourse soon after it ended.

Unlike the 1918 flu, so far COVID-19 has no massive war with which to compete in memory. And science's understanding of viruses has dramatically improved in the past century (although many COVID-19 mysteries remain). Yet, in some ways, not much has changed since our ancestors' pandemic. "Even if our experiment in lockdown, in its sheer scale and strictness, is unprecedented, we're thinking in the same way as they were" more than 100 years ago, says Laura Spinney, author of *Pale Rider: The Spanish Flu of*

1918 and How It Changed the World. "Until we have a vaccine, our main way of protecting ourselves is social distancing, and that was their main way of protecting themselves then." The current controversy about masks has a precedent, too: for instance, nearly 2,000 people attended a 1919 meeting of the Anti-Mask League of San Francisco.

Research on how political polarization affects the formation of collective memories is scant. Roediger and Wertsch suspect that divisiveness does increase the salience of an individual's recollection of an event. But Wertsch questions this effect's potential influence on a cohesive collective memory of the current pandemic. "The virus is just not an ideal character for an ideal narrative," he says.

Even the race to develop and distribute a vaccine is unlikely to yield a strong narrative, according to Wertsch. "It's conceivable that we might see a hero scientist emerge like Louis Pasteur in the 19th century," he says. "But it's noteworthy that our memory of him is precisely of him and not any particular ... epidemic." Still, with or without a strong story, COVID-19 will be much better documented than the pandemic that occurred 100 years ago. Could exhaustive media coverage strengthen a collective memory?

Media and Imagery

While the 1918 flu raged, newspapers and magazines did cover it extensively. Meg Spratt, a lecturer in communication at the University of Washington, notes that American press coverage of the pandemic prominently featured "biomilitaristic" language. Many articles framed the situation as a battle between humans (mainly government officials) and the disease. But the press of the day published "very little on the experience of the victims and survivors themselves," Spratt says. Instead coverage emphasized experts and authority–almost exclusively white men. Spratt also saw evidence that World War I overshadowed the disease. "When influenza deaths surpassed war deaths in Fall of 1918, *The New*

York Times ran the news as a small story on an inside page," she wrote in a 2001 paper on the topic.

Spratt perceives certain parallels between the coverage of the 1918 flu and that of COVID-19. "You still have this emphasis on the public health experts trying to come up with some sort of policies or recommendations to protect people," she says. "But today there seems to be this amplification. I think that comes partly from the different media technology we have." Since the Internet and social media have enabled ordinary citizens to publicly document their lives during the pandemic, Spratt says, "there's going to be richer material about what people actually went through." In this way, from firsthand accounts of essential workers to reports on racial and socioeconomic disparities in COVID-19's impacts, the media landscape of 2020 is providing a more complete picture of the current pandemic.

Photographs, too, could help to build a collective memory of COVID-19. Psychological research has consistently shown that humans' visual memory is much stronger than our recollection of words or abstract ideas. Thus, widely distributed images can form the backbone of a collective memory, Roediger says. History is filled with such iconic imagery: American troops raising the flag on Iwo Jima; the Twin Towers collapsing on 9/11; Colin Kaepernick kneeling during the national anthem. But "the cameras tend to stop at the door of the sick room or of the hospital," Spinney notes. "We tend to not go into that space." Few images show the dramatic symptoms, such as a blue face and bleeding from the ears, suffered by many who contracted the 1918 flu. Similarly, striking photographs that could reinforce collective memory are scarce in today's news reports of hospitals running over capacity, shortages of personal protective equipment and high death tolls in nursing homes.

Even if no iconic images emerge, though, individuals will certainly remember how COVID-19 affected them and their families. The same was true for the 1918 flu: in 1974 historian Richard Collier published a book compiling the personal recollections of more than 1,700 people from around the world. But as historians have discovered, collective memories ebb and flow according to the social context of the time.

Cycles of Remembering and Forgetting

This year is not the first time a new pandemic has prompted reexamination of the one in 1918. The 20th century saw two more flu pandemics, which occurred in 1957 and 1968. In both cases, "suddenly the memory of the Great Flu reoccurs," Beiner says. "People begin looking for this precedent; people begin looking for the cure." Likewise, during the avian flu scare in 2005 and the swine flu pandemic in 2009, Google searches worldwide for "Spanish flu" spiked (though both increases were dwarfed by the one that occurred this past March). All the while a growing body of historical research has been fleshing out the story of the 1918 flu, providing the foundation for a significant resurgence of its memory in the public sphere.

Beiner sees the current crisis as a tipping point in how society will remember the 1918 pandemic. Among his collection of books about it, he says, "none of them became the big novel, a book which everybody is reading. I think this might change now." Beiner predicts COVID-19 will inspire a best-selling novel or major film centered on the flu of 1918. This type of cultural landmark could serve as an anchor for public discourse about the event, fortifying the present wave of social remembering.

As for COVID-19, Beiner anticipates similar "surges in memory and then lapses in memory" over the coming decades. "We're going to have a complicated story. And it's going to always be a dialectic, dynamic forgetting and remembering working together–what happens in the public sphere and what's relegated to the private sphere," he says.

A stronger collective memory of the 1918 flu could also help create the narrative schema necessary to maintain COVID-19's public profile after today's pandemic ends. If monuments, museums or commemorations are established, they, too, would provide a social framework for continuing discussion of the current crisis. In fact, the New-York Historical Society is already collecting items related to COVID-19 for a future exhibit. "I think there will be much more impact this time because now we are aware that we didn't remember, in a public way, the Spanish flu of 1918," says José Sobral, a social anthropologist at the University of Lisbon.

Wertsch is not so sure. "In a matter of a few years," he says, "we might forget this." He suspects that how the coronavirus pandemic ends—and whether it is followed by other pandemics—will determine whether nations can weave a narrative about COVID-19 as part of a collective memory. "It's only by knowing the end," Wertsch says, "that we know the meaning of the beginning and the middle."

About the Author

Scott Hershberger was a 2020 AAAS Mass Media Fellow at Scientific American.

Lessons from Past Outbreaks Could Help Fight the Coronavirus Pandemic

By Sara Goudarzi

On March 11 the World Health Organization officially designated the novel coronavirus outbreak a pandemic. Defined as the worldwide spread of a new disease, such a declaration is the first to be made since the 2009 H1N1 swine flu. As of this writing [March 2020], there have been approximately 336,000 confirmed cases of the new disease, called COVID-19, resulting in more than 14,600 deaths worldwide.

Although a coronavirus—a family of viruses that cause illnesses ranging from the common cold to severe acute respiratory syndrome (SARS)—had not previously triggered a pandemic, this is not the first time we have seen the global transmission of a serious disease. Studying past outbreaks can help scientists better estimate the trajectory of COVID-19 and identify the best measures to slow its spread.

"Historically, we could look at everything back to the 1918 influenza pandemic. But in more contemporary times, we'd be looking at the 2015–2016 Zika outbreak in Central and South America, the global SARS outbreak from 2002 to 2003 and the Ebola outbreak in West Africa from 2014 to 2016," says Jeremy Youde, dean of the College of Liberal Arts at the University of Minnesota Duluth and an expert on global health politics.

Whereas COVID-19 is caused by a coronavirus and not an influenza virus, the 1918 flu pandemic—which caused at least 50 million deaths worldwide, according to the Centers for Disease Control and Prevention—might be the best model to understand this novel pathogen's behavior. It is also an outbreak for which massive social interventions were undertaken.

"Past influenza pandemics give some sense of what the overall [trajectory] of a virus like this would be because the reproductive number of this virus"–defined as how many people each infectious person transmits the disease to in a completely susceptible population–"is pretty similar to that of a pandemic flu," says Marc Lipsitch, a professor of epidemiology and director of the Center for Communicable Disease Dynamics at Harvard University. Although it is difficult to determine exact figures for an emerging disease, reports put the reproductive number of COVID-19 between 2 and 2.5. The median reproductive number for the 1918 flu pandemic was around 1.8. Lipsitch estimates that between about 20 and 60 percent of the global population will ultimately become infected with the novel coronavirus, or SARS-CoV-2.

Although every virus and resulting disease is different, a look at epidemic dynamics of both COVID-19 and the 1918 flu points to similar successful containment procedures. In a 2007 study published in *JAMA*, Howard Markel of the Center for the History of Medicine at the University of Michigan Medical School and his co-authors analyzed the excess deaths from pneumonia and influenza (meaning how many more there were than usual during nonpandemic years) in 43 U.S. cities from September 8, 1918 through February 22, 1919. Despite the fact that all of the cities implemented nonpharmaceutical interventions, it was the timing of activation, the duration and the combination of measures that determined their success. The researchers found "a strong association between early, sustained, and layered application of [such] interventions and mitigating the consequences of the 1918–1919 influenza pandemic in the United States."

The most effective class of nonpharmaceutical control measures were those related to social distancing: canceling public gatherings, closing places of worship, schools, bars and restaurants, isolating the sick and quarantining those they came in contact with. (Many cities around the world have adopted such measures in the current outbreak.) "In my opinion, that is probably the most important single class of things to do, as quickly as possible, to slow the spread" of a pandemic, Lipsitch says. "Waiting until you can see that you have a problem is waiting too long, because there's a delay in seeing the fruits of the measures."

By undertaking these steps early, populations can also prevent peak demands on their health care systems and flatten the pandemic curve–that is, have a gradual increase in cases over time rather than many all at once. This slowdown is especially important because it can take two or three weeks before those infected with SARS-CoV-2 are sick enough to require intensive care, so demand could spike quickly. In a 2007 *Proceedings of the National Academy of Sciences USA* paper, Lipsitch and two other researchers showed that during the 1918 influenza pandemic, cities that intervened early and intensively to slow transmission through social distancing, such as such as St. Louis, Mo., had slower epidemics with smaller peaks, compared with those that waited longer to act, such as Philadelphia.

Similarly, in a preprint report, Lipsitch and his colleagues analyzed the timing of control measures and of community spread of COVID-19 in the Chinese cities of Wuhan and Guangzhou from January 10 to February 29, 2020. Wuhan implemented measures such as strict social distancing and quarantining contacts of infected individuals six weeks after sustained local transmission was observed, whereas Guangzhou implemented these measures within one week. The researchers found that early intervention, relative to the course of the disease in the population, resulted in Guangzhou having "lower epidemic sizes and peaks" than Wuhan in the first wave of the outbreak.

Intense public measures are also one reason SARS, which resulted in around 8,000 cases with a global case fatality rate of 11 percent, was eliminated from the population. One difference, however, is that with SARS, those who were infected were likely quite sick before they became very infectious, whereas with COVID-19, people appear to be fairly infectious when they first start developing symptoms–or even before then–according to Lipsitch. In fact, in a paper published last week in *Science*, researchers note that with the novel coronavirus, "undocumented infections often experience mild, limited or no symptoms and hence go unrecognized, and, depending on their contagiousness and numbers, can expose a far greater portion of the population to virus than would otherwise occur." So despite the lower fatality rate, COVID-19 has resulted in more deaths than SARS and Middle East respiratory syndrome (MERS)–which has a 34 percent case fatality rate–combined.

Other disease countermeasures include making buildings less favorable to viral transmission by humidifying and ventilating them and implementing ongoing communication with the public so it can understand and react appropriately. One issue during the SARS outbreak was that, for a number of months, the government in China actively denied the existence of the disease. Instead people relied on text messages and rumors about a new killer flu.

"Because the government wasn't proving itself to be reliable, it became that much harder to actually address the outbreak. And it allowed the disease to really take more of a hold than it might otherwise have," Duluth's Youde says.

In order to slow down epidemics and pandemics, either the conditions for transmission need to become unfavorable over a long period of time or enough people have to become immune so that transmission cannot pick up again if the virus is reintroduced. The latter scenario, of course, means the fraction of the population that is immune has to be high enough so that each contact and infected case creates fewer than a single new one.

Regular flu and cold viruses have a strongly seasonal pattern of infectiousness in temperate regions such as the continental U.S. This seasonality is partly related to changing weather conditions and how easily the pathogens are transmitted, but it is also because of the number of susceptible hosts as people are made immune by past exposure. The same is not true of new viruses, such as the one that causes COVID-19, however.

"Pandemics happen out of season. And pandemic viruses have the whole world before them," says Lipsitch, who explains that the advantage for novel viruses is that almost no one is immune to them. Seasonal viruses, on the other hand, operate on a thinner margin–meaning the majority of people have some immunity. So those pathogens are most successful when conditions for transmission are most favorable, which is usually winter. With COVID-19, Lipsitch adds, "I think [it's] more likely seasonal changes will modestly reduce the rate of transmission and maybe slow things down–but probably not to the point of making the number of cases [decrease but rather] go up more slowly."

For now, a coordinated global effort among researchers, countries, and nongovernmental and international organizations is necessary to address the current pandemic itself while learning basic information about the virus and its spread dynamics. "In terms of having some sort of international response, we're trying to build the airplane as we're flying it," Youde says.

About the Author

Sara Goudarzi is a Brooklyn, N.Y.–based writer and author of the debut novel The Almond in the Apricot.

Stories from a Past Pandemic

By The Editors

A recent *Scientific American* feature explores how the catastrophic 1918 influenza pandemic seemed to quickly slip from public discourse. The event killed more than 50 million people worldwide, yet it takes up comparatively little space in society's "collective memory." The article considers, by analogy, how the current COVID-19 pandemic might be remembered by future generations. *Scientific American* accompanied the feature with a call for letters telling the stories of families affected by the 1918 crisis. Below are some examples of what we received.

Readers Respond

For what it's worth, and because you asked for notes about this: my grandfather died in what I believe was the second wave of the pandemic on September 24, 1918. He was 26 and otherwise very healthy. He had two daughters, aged two and under one. The older daughter was my mother, and of course, she and her sister never knew their father in any real sense. My grandmother was deeply affected by his death, as you can imagine, and she always seemed to believe that he had caught a cold and that she could have done more to save him. This made her deeply anxious, more or less permanently, about the health of everyone in the family and especially me–I was named after my grandfather and was very close to her–and I always hid any cold that I had from her. In lots of ways, my grandfather's death reverberated through the generations: it had a real effect on my mother and, eventually, me. His name was Samuel Rubinson, born August 15, 1892.

Samuel Guttenplan
Professor emeritus of philosophy,
Birkbeck, University of London

Regarding the lack of collective memory of the 1918 pandemic, I had the same question when I heard of the pandemic and that my grandmother had died during it. It was the only family story ever told about her. Gone at 38, leaving five small children. My father was nine years old. In my book, *Influenza and Inequality: One Town's Tragic Response to the Great Epidemic of 1918*, I wrote of this lack of memory. My book covers the epidemic, and epidemic behavior, in one small town–Norwood, Mass. I have dozens of personal stories in there, stories I heard from survivors, families and descendants. I believe that this lack of collective memory is linked in large part to the population of victims: the majority were young, foreign-born and poor. Influenza did not discriminate but, like today, those who could afford to stay home and avoid infection were the privileged. Then, as now, it was marginal communities–those who lived and worked in hazardous environments and lacked medical access–who were struck down. In 1918 Hispanics and Asians in California; Mexicans in New Mexico and Texas; Polish, Italian and Irish immigrants in northern cities; and, as always, Native Americans and Black individuals were the most severely affected. Children left orphaned were often adopted by others and never told of their history. And, of course, unlike today, the majority of victims were between 20 and 40 years old. Who was going to remember young, poor immigrants? Who was going to build a memorial or write a history for such outcasts? They were nameless, voiceless and, as one scholar noted, "rapidly replaced." Another early historian of the 1918 epidemic wrote, "If the pandemic had killed one or more of the really famous figures of the nation or the world it would have been remembered.... Spanish influenza characteristically killed young adults and therefore rarely men in position of great authority." That's no defense. Hopefully, today's victims will not be so invisible and easily forgotten.

Patricia J. Fanning
Professor emeritus of sociology, Bridgewater State University

I just read your article on the 1918 flu (the University of Washington sent it out on our daily newsletter because you interviewed a U.W. faculty member), and I noted the call for stories about ancestors at the end.

It's funny, that very "forgetting" rang true for me and my family, too. I just spoke with my 91-year-old grandmother about 10 days ago, and she told me that her father (my great-grandfather, Georg Monsen) survived the 1918 pandemic but that his older brother, the older brother's wife and their two kids all died of it. I've been alive for four decades and am close to my grandmother, but I never heard any of this history until now. Plus, she said that her father had hearing loss for the rest of his life because of the effects of that flu, as did other members of the family that had it but survived. This all took place in western Norway, where my grandmother is originally from.

Tabitha Grace Mallory
Henry M. Jackson School of International Studies, University of Washington

I'm 71 years old. During my college years, I'd stay at my grandmother's house almost every weekend. Grandmother and her sister, Anita, shared the house. On Sunday, we'd all go to the local Methodist church that my dad had helped build when he was younger.

One day, back home from church, my Great-Aunt Anita told me that after World War I, her whole family died from the 1918 flu: her husband and children. She believed, very strongly, that God had punished her, and she did not know why.

She still went to church and prayed.

She never talked about it again. If she'd told me how many children she'd had, I don't remember.

My Grandmother and Aunt Anita have since passed away.

Steven Oliver
via e-mail

My great-grandfather, Navy Captain John King, made it through the Great War and died of influenza on a hospital ship off City Island in New York City. My grandmother (his daughter) used to take me to lunch on City Island. We always had to drive to the end of the avenue, where we could look across the Long Island Sound and East River to where the ship had been. Grandma would recall her mother asking to be driven there to remember—remember her husband coming home from war and then being on that ship and never coming home again. After this the family (mom and four kids) moved to Baltimore, and Great-Grandma became an expert seamstress to pay the bills.

Karen Romano Young
via e-mail

Among the 675,000 people in the U.S. who lost their lives 102 years ago were nearly all of my great-grandmother's immediate family. Both of her parents and a brother died. Her first husband and their one-year-old daughter died the same day in October 1918 and were buried together in the same coffin. After losing them, she wrote a letter to the local newspaper thanking friends and neighbors for helping to see her through the devastation. At the age of only 22, she was pregnant with her second child, a son who would never know his father. She also had to raise her younger siblings who survived. Later, she remarried. I am descended from that second marriage.

This happened in Oklahoma, a state that is currently dealing with spikes of COVID-19 and very sporadic mask compliance—with no statewide mandate in place. It's demoralizing that a century after the 1918 pandemic, I have to ask: What have we learned? That those who do not learn from history are doomed to repeat it.

Shannon Leigh O'Neil
via e-mail

My dad would have been about 16 years old when the 1918 influenza both took his own father's life and sickened him. I was a child when he told me that, as the disease faded, "all [his] hair fell out." It would be interesting to know if hair loss (head, body or both) was common in survivors of that disease. I've read it can follow high fevers.

In 1920 my father—with, by then, an abundant resupply of hair—entered the U. S. Naval Academy. No doubt at least some of his classmates were also influenza survivors. I'm inclined to believe that in the process of bonding with one another, they would have shared their "collective memories" of experiencing "the flu."

It was routine, in this bonding process, for the men to confer on one another rather graphic or comic nicknames, which sometimes stuck with their recipients. I sometimes wonder whether a fellow survivor in my dad's unit, being less blessed than my dad with an exuberant regrowth of hair, gave him the nickname that would follow him for the rest of his Navy career: "Woof."

At age 75, I'm at the tail end of those who were spared by vaccination from the terrible scourges of smallpox, tetanus and diphtheria. But we had to experience for ourselves–and risk the complications–of illnesses now rarely seen in the developed world: measles, rubella, chicken pox, mumps, polio. Such experiences have certainly generated moments of collective memory.

It may not be like surviving the sinking of the *Titanic*–but each of these epidemics brought a potentially catastrophic aura, and each marked the families who suffered through them.

Elizabeth R. Hatcher
Topeka, Kan.

My paternal grandmother was born in 1900 in Conshohocken, just outside of Philadelphia, to immigrants from Molise, Italy. She was the fourth of 13 children. She was a strong women with few stories. Yet when I was a youngster in the 1960s, several times she told me a short one: "When I was 18 [years old], four of my younger [siblings] died during the [Great Influenza]. They were buried in a mass grave along the cemetery wall. My father died a few years later from a weakened heart." I am a fairly good amateur family genealogist, having uncovered many family facts, but I have been unable to track this one down well. From the local newspaper and records from the area's Catholic cemetery, I have confirmed a substantial two-week spike in deaths in Conshohocken shortly after the peak in Philadelphia in the fall. For those two weeks, the front page of the local newspaper was split vertically down the middle: one side covered the Great War, and the other side, the "Spanish flu." My great-grandfather did indeed die in 1925. For the past five decades, family stories from remote relatives only know of nine children, not 13. Unfortunately, I don't know the four other children's names or genders, as I cannot find them in the 1910 census. And by 1920 they are dead–no death certificates. I need to keep working at it.

Michael F. Iademarco
Rear admiral and assistant surgeon general,
U.S. Public Health Service

Director, Center for Surveillance,
Epidemiology, and Laboratory Services,
U.S. Centers for Disease Control and Prevention

Millions of People Living with HIV Are Alive, Thanks to a 20-Year Public Health Effort

By Lauren J. Young

After 20 years a massive U.S. government effort has reached a new milestone in its battle to defang the global HIV/AIDS epidemic: in March 2023, the Centers for Disease Control and Prevention announced that by 2022 the U.S. President's Emergency Plan for AIDS Relief (PEPFAR) had provided lifesaving antiretroviral therapy to more than 20 million people around the world with HIV—a 300-fold increase from the 66,500 people the program treated in 2004.

EPFAR's progress has shown that halting a deadly and intimidating global epidemic isn't impossible. Since the George W. Bush administration launched the ambitious plan in 2003, PEPFAR has funneled more than $110 billion into HIV/AIDS treatment and resources. It's the largest concerted public health effort by any one nation to tackle a single disease and has been credited with changing the global course of HIV/AIDS, a devastating illness that was once considered terminal.

The year PEPFAR was announced, the World Health Organization reported an estimated 40 million people were living with HIV. Countries in sub-Saharan Africa, where the epidemic was the most severe, had the majority of cases, with an estimated 26.6 million people infected. Most of Africa's health-care facilities and universities lacked resources for the testing, drug administration and monitoring needed to care for such large numbers of patients. In many parts of the continent, HIV/AIDS simply was not a survivable disease, says Phyllis Kanki, a professor of immunology and infectious diseases at Harvard University.

"We previously have had global health problems where diseases affect all populations.... But HIV was a more dramatic scourge of a pathogen because it was killing so many people, and there was no therapy," says Kanki, who helped to start the AIDS Prevention Initiative in Nigeria in 2000 and served as principal investigator for Harvard's PEPFAR program from 2004 to 2013. "I think PEPFAR has provided the solution to what was not a livable and survivable disease for scores of people who never would have had access to [HIV drugs] in the past. I think that was the big change and why it will be heralded as a huge global health success story."

Scientific American spoke with Kanki to understand how PEPFAR helped to treat millions with HIV/AIDS, how the program could inform other worldwide health crises and what stubborn barriers remain to ending the global HIV/AIDS epidemic

[An edited transcript of the interview follows.]

Q: What was the state of the HIV/AIDS epidemic in Africa in 2003?

A: In many parts of Africa, they had already been describing cases in the mid- or late 1980s. It was already appreciated at that time that there were parts of the continent that were heavily burdened, such as Botswana, South Africa–those places were already documenting 20 to 25 percent infection in the general population.

I think there was a general recognition that unlike in the U.S. and Europe, where HIV infection was mainly seen in certain risk populations (and at that time it was probably intravenous drug users and men who were having sex with men), in sub-Saharan Africa, it was a much more heterosexual, young adult population. So it was harder to target who really was at risk for being infected. That was a real concern because you didn't have good programs and infrastructure set up to rapidly diagnose these people and put them on a complex therapy even if that therapy was available to you.

There was a lot of variability on the continent, but generally there weren't many accessible programs for people to receive drugs if they found out they were infected with HIV. Those with means who found out they were positive might have to pay huge sums of money to get drugs or go to Europe or the U.S. for treatment. But that was certainly just a small proportion. There were not known government programs that were readily set up to help people. And that was particularly true in places that were hardest hit and had what was already known to be the largest proportion of infected individuals.

Q: Why was PEPFAR started?

A: As a minimum standard of care, you have to have a good diagnosis; you have to be able to bring in the drugs–the drugs all have to be there; you have to give the treatment to patients every month; you have to have a system so you know you're giving it to them; and then you have to have a way of monitoring them. And none of that was in place.

One of the reasons it was such a challenge for people in international health to grapple with HIV is that it was such a complicated disease. It's hard to diagnose. You can't treat somebody if you don't know they have it. Then once you put somebody on treatment, it's lifelong. At the time, patients were having to take six to 12 pills once, twice, three times a day. And it's absolutely critical that they take the pills every day because if they stopped, the viruses that are still in their bodies would become active again, and they can get sick and could die. Some pills require refrigeration. Some pills you couldn't take unless you had already eaten a meal. In some of our clinics, if populations were food-insecure, we had to provide food. And you have to monitor people with tests that most of the labs or university hospital facilities didn't have the equipment for. Who was going to pay for these tests? You couldn't ask patients to pay, and you couldn't ask labs that didn't have the equipment to run the test.

We also had problems in some populations in Africa where there was a lot of comorbidity–another disease you see with HIV is tuberculosis [TB], which a real killer all by itself. You had to deal with managing two different therapies for two different complex diseases.

Around that time, the government of Nigeria had tried to purchase generic drugs in India to provide treatment for some of the first HIV-infected individuals, recognizing it had a huge population that was already infected. They started the government program, but it was very small. Governments in Africa had already tried to begin these programs, but PEPFAR was a shot in the arm. We were able to use PEPFAR funds to really bolster what was just the beginning of Nigeria's program.

Today PEPFAR works in more than 50 countries, providing health-care infrastructure and resources–including antiretroviral therapy (ART)–to stymie the spread of HIV. What is ART, and how has it transformed HIV/AIDS care?

The virus itself enters a key cell that's important in defending your body from outside pathogens, and that cell is the lymphocyte. It's one of your white blood cells that circulates through your body and in certain organs. It's a key player in protecting you. So one of the villainous properties of the virus is that it integrates; it inserts its genetic material into yours. And that's why an infection with a retrovirus such as HIV is forever–because you can't get rid of it.

There are different classes of ART drugs that operate on different parts of the virus's life cycle. Some will basically stop the virus before it integrates. Other drugs inhibit the integration step. Others block the virus's entry into cells.

When we started out, we showed slides of people with two hands together with a pile of pills. Currently it's probably one pill a day–that's a single pill that includes multiple drugs. Those pills are much more effective than what we were able to give out before. So things have really changed in 20 years.

Q: What's on the horizon for HIV/AIDS treatments?

A: There's PrEP (pre-exposure prophylaxis): if you're uninfected, this pill will help prevent you from being infected by another individual. There are different modalities and ways we would use these very effective therapies to try to limit spread or to decrease virus so that people don't get sick. There's a continued effort to develop a vaccine.

There's a lot of research being done on what's called the HIV cure [a few people reportedly have been cleared of HIV or considered to be in long-term remission after receiving HIV-resistant stem cells] and different ways that researchers think they can try to get rid of the disease. But certainly that's still a work in progress, I'd say.

Q: What disparities and stigma still exist around HIV/AIDS? What efforts are there to identify those who need treatment and make sure they can access it?

A: There's stigma with a lot of different diseases, but we see in Africa that people don't want to be known to have HIV infection, because maybe it carries the stigma that they had multiple sex partners or had used drugs. Even just that you're not healthy–that can be a stigma in certain populations.

We've been involved with projects for men who have sex with men in Nigeria, and that's a very stigmatized population. It's very hard for them to identify and find supportive clinics, which are quasi-underground, to be able to get access to the care. That's partially because there are laws in those countries that criminalize their sexual orientation.

Africa has the largest number of kids who were infected at birth. Those kids are growing up, and many of them are stigmatized–they're 12 years old, and they've just been told by their mother that they've been taking pills, and those pills are for HIV. They don't want their classmates or other people in the community to know that's what they have because it reflects badly on them and also on their family. So then they don't want to go to the clinic and be seen. We do have problems with adolescents when they're grappling with a lot of other issues in their life and having to deal with the fact that they're supposed to go to a clinic every month that identifies them as having HIV. They're going to have to do that for the rest of their life.

Q: What do you think are the major next steps to reaching PEPFAR's goal of ending the HIV/AIDS epidemic as a public health threat by 2030? How realistic is it?

A: A lot of these international goals are kind of pies in the sky, but you have to keep going. You can't stop when you're 10 feet from the goal line. Many countries are very close to providing treatment to every person with HIV. I think Botswana, for example, is very close. It has a large infected population but has been very successful in identifying and treating all the people who are affected. And the goals to prevent infection and to treat every pregnant woman who's positive can really make a difference in getting rid of infant HIV infection because that's a starting point.

Q: What lessons from PEPFAR could be applied to other epidemics or disease-prevention strategies?

A: It was a brand-new approach to a global health problem. I think PEPFAR was different because it committed such a large amount of money to one disease, primarily in parts of the world that were most affected—those that were the poorest parts that would not have been able to do anything at that time with what was available. PEPFAR was really the ambulance with the medicine. The size of it and the scope of it were so huge. Those of us who were working in Africa were kind of amazed at the idea that a U.S. program would commit so much money to people in Africa. We were happy about it, of course. We had never seen anything like it. So it was really a tremendous opportunity, and no one knew whether it would really work. And 20 years later we see that it did. It really made a huge difference for health care overall, not just HIV care, in all of these countries.

AIDS is caused by one virus, but it affects other things such as TB. So I do think the PEPFAR program provided a lot of important lessons for how we could deal with the Global TB Program. It did bolster the infrastructure that was available for TB, and it certainly improved care for that. Many of the labs that were developed for providing HIV services have been used for things such as Ebola and mpox. I think all of that has a trickle-down effect of improving health-care services overall.

And that's why I think PEPFAR will be recognized for many additional benefits that are outside of just dealing with the horrible issue of the HIV pandemic and AIDS. Many other health-care problems were addressed on the side. We're in a better position to deal with HIV than we were in 2004, for sure.

About the Author

Lauren J. Young is an associate editor for health and medicine at Scientific American.

HIV Care Has Improved Dramatically—But Not for Everyone

By David Malebranche

On a sweltering June day in 2021, Nicole, whose real name has been changed to protect her privacy, walked into an HIV treatment clinic in Atlanta, Ga., expecting something different. She had shouldered a lifetime of discrimination for being both Black and transgender while also dealing with HIV, diabetes and hypertension. She worked as a manager of a fast-food restaurant while parenting several LGBTQ youths. Accessing consistent health care was a daily battle, and Nicole's past interactions with providers had left her feeling discouraged. But she and I had hit it off during a previous telemedicine appointment, so she scheduled a face-to-face visit at the clinic where I worked. As a Black, same-gender-loving physician, I wanted to do better by her.

Despite the amazing scientific advances in HIV care that have taken place since the epidemic began 40 years ago, many people in racially and sexually minoritized communities still fall through the cracks. Some can't afford care, and others can't access it because of job or family demands, lack of transportation or documentation, or other barriers. Many face stigma and discrimination from medical providers themselves. I was determined to do everything I could to change the narrative of Nicole's health-care experiences that day.

She obtained HIV medications through the AIDS Drug Assistance Program, which provides antiretroviral therapy (ART) for the uninsured. To remain eligible for the state-sponsored program, she endured cumbersome bureaucratic paperwork, drove 45 minutes each way to the clinic for regular visits and attended required meetings with a benefits counselor every six months. To save money, she filled prescriptions for some of her other conditions at several different local pharmacies. She got her hormones off the street because a previous clinician had refused to prescribe them unless she sought mental health counseling first.

Nicole arrived 30 minutes late for our appointment after a long commute into the city during rush-hour traffic. As we discussed her gender identity, sexual health and romantic partners, I saw a surprised look on her face, suggesting to me that few clinicians had asked her these questions before. Her physical exam was mostly normal, except for extensive anal warts. "They've been there a long time," she said. "No one knows what to do with them." I imagined some medical providers being so uncomfortable with her being transgender that they bypassed the genital exam altogether.

As we sat together in that sterile exam room, I realized that the medical community had failed her, and it wasn't because of a lack of advances in HIV treatment and prevention. ART has evolved from toxic medications taken multiple times a day to single-tablet regimens with few side effects. We now have bimonthly injections that can maintain full viral suppression. First approved in 2012, preexposure prophylaxis, or PrEP, given as a daily oral pill or bimonthly injection can reduce one's chances of contracting HIV by 90 to 100 percent. Despite these great scientific strides, Nicole wasn't reaping the benefits of this progress.

What's to blame? Many social, institutional and interpersonal medical barriers are. Inequities in housing and food insecurity, access to insurance, and bias and stigma in medical care contribute to persistent racial and ethnic disparities in HIV incidence rates, engagement in care and viral suppression. For Nicole, HIV is just one of many circumstances that make everyday life challenging. America's fragmented and dysfunctional health-care system only makes things worse.

These disparate HIV health outcomes are complicated by a labyrinth of bureaucracy within medical spaces that make it nearly impossible for many to access medications that should be within their reach. This includes cumbersome paperwork to obtain ART if one is uninsured, underresourced clinics and medical staff burnt out from COVID, and institutional policies that prioritize visit numbers and copay billing over patient-centered care. For people living with HIV, these issues within our nation's clinics can make getting and staying on ART a climb that feels insurmountable.

After her exam, Nicole asked, "So, can I get my lab work done?" Unfortunately, because our appointment started late, the technicians had already left for the day. She would have to make another trip. Even our clinic, which worked hard to help those who needed it most, wasn't flexible enough to help her on this occasion. As I watched her face cloud with disappointment, I feared we would lose her again. I feared that I was failing her, like so many clinicians before me.

Despite my concerns, Nicole told me she left that day feeling encouraged because she felt heard for the first time in eons. We planned to restart her ART, refer her to colorectal surgery to evaluate her warts, explore insurance options with her employer and consolidate all her medications at a single pharmacy. I sent in her hormone prescriptions, confirming what she already knew: there is no universal policy requiring a mental health specialist to approve them.

The burden of improving HIV prevention and treatment is now on the shoulders of our medical systems. As we seek to provide more equitable care, statewide and national policy improvements must be accompanied by changes within health-care systems and clinics: We must enhance case management staff to ensure patients can get to their appointments and understand the processes required to access treatment. We must make sure patients can have necessary blood work done on the day of their checkup appointment. We must develop sensible patient-flow protocols to ensure that people are seen in a timely and efficient manner. Offering patients a diverse range of appointments, such as telehealth, walk-ins and house calls, can accommodate the fluidity of life. Clinics need to hire staff and providers who reflect the communities served, and they should invest in cultural humility training to reduce bias and stigma in treatment. Modifications at the clinic level, though relatively small compared with sweeping national policies, can have an enormous impact on whether someone living with HIV decides to continue accessing care there or not.

Medical approaches to HIV prevention and treatment have come a long way. These revolutionary breakthroughs can help tackle the current HIV health inequities in the U.S. and ultimately lead to a cure. But this will all be for naught if the medical systems and personnel who are the gatekeepers to these advances act more like health-care barriers than facilitators.

I'd like to tell you that the work we did that day helped Nicole feel more optimistic about trusting medical systems and providers. I'd like to tell you that her future clinic appointments went smoothly and didn't require repeat visits. I'd like to tell you that she found her voice with her employer, obtained private insurance through her job and is now receiving care for all her medical issues. I'd like to tell you she is being treated by other medical staff with the dignity and respect she deserves.

But I can't. She missed our next appointment, and by the time the clinic was able to reschedule her, I had stopped working there. Truth is, patients fall out of care more often than we like to admit, sometimes because of a revolving door of clinical providers entering and leaving these settings. I took solace in knowing that we had connected that day and that I did my best to give her the medical care she deserved. Perhaps our interaction restored her faith in human connectedness–a dynamic that may alleviate some of the harm inflicted by broken and discriminatory health-care systems. Nicole came to our appointment expecting something different. I hope she now realizes that something different is possible.

About the Author

David Malebranche is an internal medicine physician with 20 years of clinical and public health expertise in sexual health and HIV/STI treatment and prevention. He resides in Atlanta, Ga.

Lessons from AIDS for the COVID-19 Pandemic

By William A. Haseltine

We are now engaged in another deadly episode in the historic battle of man versus microbe. These battles have shaped the course of human evolution and of history. We have seen the face of our adversary, in this case a tiny virus." I spoke these words in testimony before a U.S. Senate subcommittee on September 26, 1985. I was talking about HIV, but I could say the same thing today about the coronavirus we are facing.

Like all viruses, coronaviruses are expert code crackers. SARS-CoV-2 has certainly cracked ours. Think of this virus as an intelligent biological machine continuously running DNA experiments to adapt to the ecological niche it inhabits. This virus has caused a pandemic in large part because it acted on three of our most human vulnerabilities: our biological defenses, our clustering patterns of social behavior and our simmering political divides.

How will the confrontation unfold in the next years and decades? What will be the human toll in deaths, ongoing disease, injuries and other impairments? How effective will new vaccines and treatments be in containing or even eradicating the virus?

No one can say. But several lessons from the long battle with HIV, the human immunodeficiency virus that causes AIDS, suggest what may lie ahead. HIV/AIDS is one of the worst scourges humans have encountered. As a code cracker, HIV is an expert. By the end of 2019 the global death toll from this virus was roughly 33 million people. In all, 76 million people have been infected, and scientists estimate another 1.7 million people acquire the virus every year.

Yet we must appreciate what our scientific defenses have accomplished. Of the nearly 38 million people currently living with HIV/AIDS, 25 million are receiving full antiretroviral treatments that prevent disease and suppress the virus so well they are unlikely to pass it along. I would wager that another 25 million or more infections never happened, primarily in sub-Saharan Africa, because these treatments became available in most countries.

From fighting this epic war against AIDS, doctors, virologists, epidemiologists and public health experts have learned crucial lessons that we can apply to the battle we are currently waging. For instance, we saw that vaccines are never a guarantee but that treatments can be our most important weapon. We discovered that human behavior plays a vital role in any disease-fighting effort and that we cannot overlook human nature. We have also seen how critical it is to build on knowledge and tools gained fighting earlier outbreaks–a strategy only possible if we continue funding research in between pandemics.

Vaccine Challenges

Early observations of how HIV behaves in our bodies showed the road to a vaccine would be long and challenging. As the outbreak unfolded, we began tracking antibody levels and T cells (the white blood cells that wage war against invaders) in those infected. The high levels of both showed that patients were mounting incredibly active immune responses, more forceful than anything we had seen for any other disease. But even working at its highest capacity, the body's immune system was never strong enough to clear out the virus completely.

Unlike the hit-and-run polio virus, which evokes long-term immunity after an infection, HIV is a "catch it and keep it" virus–if you are infected, the pathogen stays in your body until it destroys the immune system, leaving you undefended against even mild infections. Moreover, HIV continually evolves–a shrewd opponent seeking ways to elude our immune responses. Although this does not mean a vaccine is impossible, it certainly meant developing one, especially when the virus hit in the 1980s, would not be easy. "Unfortunately, no one can predict with certainty that an AIDS vaccine can ever be made," I testified in 1988 to the Presidential

Commission on the HIV Epidemic. "That is not to say it is impossible to make such a vaccine, only that we are not certain of success." More than 30 years later there still is no effective vaccine to prevent HIV infection.

From what we have seen of SARS-CoV-2, it interacts with our immune system in complex ways, resembling polio in some of its behavior and HIV in others. We know from nearly 60 years of observing coronaviruses that a body's immune system can clear them. That seems to be generally the case for SARS-CoV-2 as well. But the cold-causing coronaviruses, just like HIV, also have their tricks. Infection from one of them never seems to confer immunity to reinfection or symptoms by the same strain of virus—that is why the same cold viruses return each season. These coronaviruses are not a hit-and-run virus like polio or a catch-it-and-keep-it virus like HIV. I call them "get it and forget it" viruses—once cleared, your body tends to forget it ever fought this foe. Early studies with SARS-CoV-2 suggest it might behave much like its cousins, raising transient immune protection.

The path to a SARS-CoV-2 vaccine may be filled with obstacles. Whereas some people with COVID-19 make neutralizing antibodies that can clear the virus, not everybody does. Whether a vaccine will stimulate such antibodies in everyone is still unknown. Moreover, we do not know how long those antibodies can protect someone from infection. It may be two or three years before we will have the data to tell us and any confidence in the outcome.

Another challenge is how this virus enters the body: through the nasal mucosal membranes. No COVID-19 vaccine currently in development has shown an ability to prevent infection through the nose. In nonhuman primates, some vaccines can prevent the disease from spreading efficiently to the lungs. But those studies do not tell us much about how the same drug will work in humans; the disease in our species is very different from what it is in monkeys, which do not become noticeably ill.

We learned with HIV that attempts to prevent virus entry altogether do not work well—not for HIV and not for many other viruses, including influenza and even polio. Vaccines act more like fire alarms: rather than preventing fires from breaking out, they call the immune system for help once a fire has ignited.

The hopes of the world rest on a COVID-19 vaccine. It seems likely that scientists will announce a "success" sometime this year, but success is not as simple as it sounds. As I write, officials in Russia have reported approving a COVID-19 vaccine. Will it work? Will it be safe? Will it be long lasting? No one will be able to provide convincing answers to these questions for any forthcoming vaccine soon, perhaps not for at least several years.

We have made remarkable improvements in our molecular biology tools since the 1980s, yet the slowest part of drug development remains human testing. That said, the infrastructure created for HIV/AIDS research is accelerating the testing process now. Thirty thousand volunteers around the world participate in networks built by the National Institutes of Health for studies of new HIV vaccine candidates, and these networks are being tapped for initial testing of COVID-19 vaccines, too.

When doctors treat a patient who is likely to die, they are willing to risk that a drug might sicken the patient but still save their life. But doctors are less willing to do that to *prevent* disease; the chances of causing greater harm to the patient are too high. This is why for decades the quest for a vaccine to prevent HIV infection has lagged so far behind development of therapeutic drugs for HIV.

Focus on Treatments

These drugs now stand as an incredible success story.

The first set of HIV drugs were nucleic acid inhibitors, known as chain terminator drugs. They inserted an additional "chain terminating" nucleotide as the virus copied its viral RNA into DNA, preventing the HIV chain of DNA from elongating.

By the 1990s we had gotten better at using combinations of drugs to control HIV infections soon after patients were exposed. The first drug, AZT, found immediate application for health care workers who accidentally had a needlestick injury that infected them with contaminated blood. It was also used to reduce mother-to-child transmission. For example, prenatal treatments for mothers with AIDS at that time reduced the number of babies born infected by as much as two thirds. Today combination chemotherapy reduces mother-to-child transmission to undetectable levels.

The next set of drugs was protease inhibitors, one of which I helped to develop. The first was introduced in 1995 and was combined with other drugs in treating patients. These drugs inhibited the viral protease enzyme responsible for longer precursor proteins in the short active components of the virus. But there is a fundamental problem with these drugs, as well as those that inhibit viral polymerases, which help to create virus DNA. Our bodies also use proteases for normal functioning, and we need polymerases to replicate our own nucleic acids. The same drugs that inhibit the viral proteins also inhibit our own cells. The difference between a concentration in which the drug inhibits the virus target and a concentration in which it hurts the human proteins is called the therapeutic index. The therapeutic index gives you the window in which the drug will be effective against the virus without causing undue side effects. That window is rather narrow for all polymerase and protease inhibitors.

The gold standard for AIDS treatment now is called antiretroviral therapy—essentially patients take a cocktail of at least three different drugs that attack the HIV virus in different ways. The strategy is based on earlier success we had in fighting cancer. In the late 1970s I established a laboratory at Harvard University's Dana-Farber Cancer Institute to develop new drugs to treat cancer patients. Cancers developed resistance over time to single drugs, but combinations of drugs were effective in slowing, stopping or killing the cancers. We took that same lesson of combination chemotherapy to HIV. By the early 1990s the first combination AIDS treatments were saving the lives of people infected with HIV. Today an infection is far from the death sentence it used to be—patients can now live almost unaffected by HIV, with a relatively minimal impact on life expectancy.

We already know resistance to single drugs will bedevil COVID-19 treatments. We have seen resistance to single, anti-SARS-CoV-2 drugs develop rapidly in early lab studies. Just as with AIDS and cancer, we need a combination of medicines to treat this disease. The goal of the biotechnology and pharmaceutical industries now is to develop an array of highly potent and specific drugs, each of which targets a different function of the virus. Decades of research on HIV has shown the way and gives us confidence in our eventual success.

Human Behavior

In trying to understand and counter the AIDS epidemic, physician and virologist Robert Redfield (who is now head of the Centers for Disease Control and Prevention) and I became good friends in the early 1980s. We quickly learned that while many politicians across the globe refused to recognize HIV as a threat to their populations, militaries were an exception. Nearly all countries considered AIDS a serious danger to troops and military readiness and a potentially huge drain on future military funds. Their view was, "Let's not blind ourselves and pretend soldiers are saints. They are not. They are humans." Redfield, then at Walter Reed Army Medical Center, helped to design and manage a program to test the entire U.S. uniformed forces for HIV infection (although the consequences of this test were controversial, and recruits who tested positive were barred from service).

At the time there were no effective drugs; the disease killed more than 90 percent of those infected. When married couples were tested and one partner was infected and one not, doctors advised them in the strongest possible terms to use condoms. I was stunned to learn that fewer than a third complied with the advice. "If people don't respond to the lethal danger of unprotected sex with their husband or wife, we are in real trouble," I thought. Over the next five years more than three quarters of the uninfected partners contracted HIV.

I have always used this experience as a guide to pit hope against reality. Human sexuality–the drive for sex and physical connection–

is deeply embedded in our nature. I knew in the 1980s it was very unlikely people would change their sexual behavior in a major way. In the 19th century everyone knew how syphilis was contracted and that it was serious disease. Yet syphilis still infected at least 10 to 15 percent of American citizens at the beginning of the 20th century. It was not that people were ignorant of how to catch it; it is that they did not change their lifestyle accordingly.

There is likewise a sexual dynamic to COVID-19 that often goes unmentioned. It is part of what is driving people out of their homes and into bars and parties. Anyone with a craving for a beer can quench their thirst in the safety of their own home, but gratification comes less easily for other desires, especially when one is young, single and living alone. Our public health strategies should not ignore this fact.

The same lessons we learned in the midst of the HIV epidemic to help young people change their behaviors apply today to COVID-19: know your risk, know your partners and take necessary precautions. Many young people operate under the false assumption that even if they become infected, they will not become severely ill. Not only is this belief untrue, but even people with asymptomatic infections can suffer serious, lasting damage. But the more people understand the risk–younger people especially–the greater likelihood they will take the steps necessary to protect themselves and others. We saw this happen with AIDS.

Funding

When I ask world experts what they know about the detailed molecular biology of SARS-CoV-2 or, for that matter, any other coronavirus, they do not have the kind of answers they should. Why? Because governments and industry pulled the plug on coronavirus research funding in 2006 after the first SARS (severe acute respiratory syndrome) pandemic faded away and again in the years immediately following the MERS (Middle East respiratory syndrome, also caused by a coronavirus) outbreak when it seemed to be controllable. Funding agencies everywhere, not just in the U.S. but in China, Japan, Singapore, Hong Kong and the Middle East–countries affected by SARS and MERS–underestimated the threat of coronaviruses. Despite clear, persistent, highly vocal warnings from many of those who battled SARS and MERS up close, funding dried up. The development of promising anti-SARS and MERS drugs, which might have been active against SARS-CoV-2 as well, was left unfinished for lack of money.

With 776,000 dead and 22 million infected globally as of mid-August, we have every motive to accelerate funding. The U.S. quickly opened the funding spigots last spring for research to hasten discoveries of vaccines and drugs. But will it be enough?

We learned from the HIV crisis that it was important to have research pipelines already established. Cancer research in the 1950s, 1960s and 1970s built a foundation for HIV/AIDS studies. The government responded to public concerns, sharply increasing federal funding of cancer research during those decades. These efforts culminated in Congress's approval of President Richard Nixon's National Cancer Act in 1971. This $1.6-billion commitment for cancer research, equal to $10 billion in today's money, built the science we needed to identify and understand HIV in the 1980s, although of course no one knew that payoff was coming.

In the 1980s the Reagan administration did not want to talk about AIDS or commit much public funding to HIV research. The first time President Ronald Reagan gave a major speech on AIDS was in 1987. In his first administration, funding for HIV research was scarce; few scientists were willing to stake their careers on deciphering the molecular biology. Yet once the news broke that actor Rock Hudson was seriously ill with AIDS, Ted Stevens, the Senate Republican Whip, joined with Democratic Senator Ted Kennedy, actor Elizabeth Taylor, me and a few others in campaigning effectively to add $320 million in the fiscal 1986 budget for AIDS research. Barry Goldwater, Jesse Helms and John Warner, Republican leaders in the Senate, supported us. The money flowed, and outstanding scientists signed on. I helped to design this first congressionally funded AIDS research program with Anthony Fauci, the doctor now leading our nation's fight against COVID-19. (And if there is one person in the world who has made the greatest contribution to the prevention and treatment of AIDS, that person is Fauci.)

One difference between the 1980s and now is that Republican members of Congress were more willing to stand up to the president and White House staff when they failed to take the necessary steps to fight a global disease. For example, Stevens decided it was his job to protect the U.S. Army and other arms of the military and Secret Service as much as possible from HIV infection. He helped to move $55 million within the defense budget, designating it for screening recruits for HIV/AIDS.

Our tool set for virus and pharmaceutical research has improved enormously in the past 36 years since HIV was discovered. This is one reason I am confident we will have effective antiviral drugs for treating COVID-19 infections by next year, if not sooner. What used to take us five or 10 years in the 1980s and 1990s in many cases now can be done in five or 10 months. We can rapidly identify and synthesize chemicals to predict which drugs will be effective. We can do cryoelectron microscopy to probe virus structures and simulate molecule-by-molecule interactions in a matter of weeks—something that used to take years. The lesson is to never let down our guard when it comes to funding antivirus research. We would have no hope of beating COVID-19 if it were not for the molecular biology gains we made during earlier virus battles. What we learn this time around will help us out during the next pandemic, but we must keep the money coming.

A Leap into Darkness

In November 2019 I spent several days in Wuhan, China, chairing a meeting of the U.S.-China Health Summit. Our group's major concern, looming amid the U.S.-China trade war, was the threat of restrictions on sharing research discoveries. Otherwise, it was a delightful time in a beautiful city.

Weeks later, back home in New York City, I could not shake a lingering cold virus infection I picked up on the Wuhan trip. (I later tested negative for COVID-19 antibodies, but that result is not definitive.) The head of my foundation in China called me one day with awful news. Three of his grandparents had died from some strange virus. "Everyone who gets this is really sick," my colleague, in his mid-30s, said. "Everything is closed down. I can't even go to my grandparents' funerals."

A few weeks later I received a vivid firsthand account of how aggressively China was confronting the outbreak from another colleague who had just emerged from 14 days of isolation in a quarantine hotel. He explained that when one person in the back of his flight from Frankfurt, Germany, to Shanghai tested positive for the coronavirus, contact tracers called my friend days later and ordered him into isolation. His only human contact then was with hazmat-clad inspectors who came daily to disinfect his room and drop off meals.

We are just beginning to glimpse what the long-term toll of COVID-19 might be. This is a new virus, so we will not have a clearer idea until after a few years, but we know it will be very high. We have *barely* scratched the surface of coronavirus molecular biology. What story will our children and grandchildren recount about our successes as scientists and as a society, and our failures, to contain this pandemic–the worst we have faced in 100 years?

Science leaps into the darkness, the very edge of human knowledge. That is where we begin, as if deep in a cave, chipping away at a wall of hard stone. You do not know what you will find on the other side. Some people chip away for a lifetime, only to accumulate a pile of flakes. We may be in for a protracted pandemic, or we may get lucky with effective treatments and vaccines soon. But we have been here before, facing an unknown viral enemy, and we can lean on lessons we have learned. This is not the first and will not be the last global epidemic.

About the Author

William A. Haseltine is a former Harvard Medical School professor and founder of the university's cancer and HIV/AIDS research departments. He also serves as chair and president of the global health think tank ACCESS Health International. He has founded more than a dozen biotechnology companies and is the author, most recently, of Variants! The Shape-Shifting Challenge of COVID-19.

Section 2: The Science and Medicine of COVID-19

2.1 How China's 'Bat Woman' Hunted Down Viruses from SARS to the New Coronavirus
By Jane Qiu

2.2 A High-Speed Scientific Hive Mind Emerged from the COVID Pandemic
By Joseph Bak-Coleman and Carl T. Bergstrom

2.3 An mRNA Pioneer Discusses How Her Work Led to the COVID Vaccines
By Tanya Lewis

2.4 Messenger RNA Therapies Are Finally Fulfilling Their Promise
By Drew Weissman

2.5 Pandemic-Era Research Will Pay Off for Years
By Britt Glaunsinger

2.6 COVID Revealed the Fragility of American Public Health
By Wendy E. Parmet

2.7 COVID Pushed Global Health Institutions to Their Limits
By Lawrence O. Gostin

How China's 'Bat Woman' Hunted Down Viruses from SARS to the New Coronavirus

By Jane Qiu

The mysterious patient samples arrived at the Wuhan Institute of Virology at 7 P.M. on December 30, 2019. Moments later Shi Zhengli's cell phone rang. It was her boss, the institute's director. The Wuhan Center for Disease Control and Prevention had detected a novel coronavirus in two hospital patients with atypical pneumonia, and it wanted Shi's renowned laboratory to investigate. If the finding was confirmed, the new pathogen could pose a serious public health threat—because it belonged to the same family of viruses as the one that caused severe acute respiratory syndrome (SARS), a disease that plagued 8,100 people and killed nearly 800 of them between 2002 and 2003. "Drop whatever you are doing and deal with it now," she recalls the director saying.

Shi, a virologist who is often called China's "bat woman" by her colleagues because of her virus-hunting expeditions in bat caves over the past 16 years, walked out of the conference she was attending in Shanghai and hopped on the next train back to Wuhan. "I wondered if [the municipal health authority] got it wrong," she says. "I had never expected this kind of thing to happen in Wuhan, in central China." Her studies had shown that the southern, subtropical provinces of Guangdong, Guangxi and Yunnan have the greatest risk of coronaviruses jumping to humans from animals—particularly bats, a known reservoir. If coronaviruses were the culprit, she remembers thinking, "Could they have come from our lab?"

While Shi's team at the Wuhan institute, an affiliate of the Chinese Academy of Sciences, raced to uncover the identity of the contagion—over the following week they connected the illness to the novel coronavirus that become known as SARS-CoV-2—the disease spread like wildfire. By April 20 more than 84,000 people in China had been infected. About 80 percent of them lived in the province of Hubei, of which Wuhan is the capital, and more than 4,600 had died. Outside of China, about 2.4 million people across 210 or so countries and territories had caught the virus, and more than 169,000 had perished from the disease it caused, COVID-19.

Scientists have long warned that the rate of emergence of new infectious diseases is accelerating—especially in developing countries where high densities of people and animals increasingly mingle and move about. "It's incredibly important to pinpoint the source of infection and the chain of cross-species transmission," says disease ecologist Peter Daszak, president of EcoHealth Alliance, a New York City–based nonprofit research organization that collaborates with researchers, such as Shi, in 30 countries in Asia, Africa and the Middle East to discover new viruses in wildlife. An equally important task, he adds, is to hunt down other pathogens to "prevent similar incidents from happening again."

The Caves

To Shi, her first virus-discovery expedition felt like a vacation. On a breezy, sunny spring day in 2004, she joined an international team of researchers to collect samples from bat colonies in caves near Nanning, the capital of Guangxi. Her inaugural cave was typical of the region: large, rich in limestone columns and—as a popular tourist destination—easily accessible. "It was spellbinding," Shi recalls. Milky-white stalactites hung from the ceiling like icicles, glistening with moisture.

But the holiday-like atmosphere soon dissipated. Many bats—including several insect-eating species of horseshoe bats that are abundant in southern Asia—roost in deep, narrow caves on steep terrain. Often guided by tips from local villagers, Shi and her colleagues had to hike for hours to potential sites and inch through tight rock crevasses on their stomachs. And the flying mammals can be elusive. In one frustrating week, the team explored more than 30 caves and saw only a dozen bats.

These expeditions were part of the effort to catch the culprit in the SARS outbreak, the first major epidemic of the 21st century. A Hong Kong team had reported that wildlife traders in Guangdong first caught the SARS coronavirus from civets, mongooselike mammals that are native to tropical and subtropical Asia and Africa.

Before SARS, the world had only an inkling of coronaviruses—so named because their spiky surface resembles a crown when seen under a microscope, says Linfa Wang, who directs the emerging infectious diseases program at Singapore's Duke-NUS Medical School. Coronaviruses were mostly known for causing common colds. "The SARS outbreak was a game changer," Wang says. It was the first emergence of a deadly coronavirus with pandemic potential. The incident helped to jump-start a global search for animal viruses that could find their way into humans. Shi was an early recruit of that effort, and both Daszak and Wang have been her long-term collaborators.

With the SARS virus, just how the civets got it remained a mystery. Two previous incidents were telling: Australia's 1994 Hendra virus infections, in which the contagion jumped from horses to humans, and Malaysia's 1998 Nipah virus outbreak, in which it moved from pigs to people. Wang found that both diseases were caused by pathogens that originated in fruit-eating bats. Horses and pigs were merely the intermediate hosts. Bats in the Guangdong market also contained traces of the SARS virus, but many scientists dismissed this as contamination. Wang, however, thought bats might be the source.

In those first virus-hunting months in 2004, whenever Shi's team located a bat cave, it would put a net at the opening before dusk and then wait for the nocturnal creatures to venture out to feed for the night. Once the bats were trapped, the researchers took blood and saliva samples, as well as fecal swabs, often working into the small hours. After catching up on some sleep, they would return to the cave in the morning to collect urine and fecal pellets.

But sample after sample turned up no trace of genetic material from coronaviruses. It was a heavy blow. "Eight months of hard work seemed to have gone down the drain," Shi says. "We thought maybe bats had nothing to do with SARS." The scientists were about to give up when a research group in a neighboring lab handed them a diagnostic kit for testing antibodies produced by people with SARS.

There was no guarantee that the test would work for bat antibodies, but Shi gave it a go anyway. "What did we have to lose?" she says. The results exceeded her expectations. Samples from three horseshoe bat species contained antibodies to the SARS virus. "It was a turning point for the project," Shi says. The researchers learned that the presence of the coronavirus in bats was ephemeral and seasonal–but an antibody reaction could last from weeks to years. The diagnostic kit, therefore, offered a valuable pointer as to how to hunt down viral genomic sequences.

Shi's team used the antibody test to narrow down the list of locations and bat species to pursue in the quest for genomic clues. After roaming mountainous terrain in most of China's dozens of provinces, the researchers turned their attention to one spot: Shitou Cave, on the outskirts of Kunming, the capital of Yunnan, where they conducted intense sampling during different seasons over five consecutive years.

The efforts paid off. The pathogen hunters discovered hundreds of bat-borne coronaviruses with incredible genetic diversity. "The majority of them are harmless," Shi says. But dozens belong to the same group as SARS. They can infect human lung cells in a petri dish and cause SARS-like diseases in mice.

In Shitou Cave–where painstaking scrutiny has yielded a natural genetic library of bat-borne viruses–the team discovered a coronavirus strain that came from horseshoe bats with a genomic sequence nearly 97 percent identical to the one found in civets in Guangdong. The finding concluded a decade-long search for the natural reservoir of the SARS coronavirus.

A Dangerous Mix

In many bat dwellings Shi has sampled, including Shitou Cave, "constant mixing of different viruses creates a great opportunity for dangerous new pathogens to emerge," says Ralph Baric, a virologist at the University of North Carolina at Chapel Hill. In the vicinity of such viral melting pots, Shi says, "you don't need to be a wildlife trader to be infected."

Near Shitou Cave, for example, many villages sprawl among the lush hillsides in a region known for its roses, oranges, walnuts and hawthorn berries. In October 2015 Shi's team collected blood samples from more than 200 residents in four of those villages. It found that six people, or nearly 3 percent, carried antibodies against SARS-like coronaviruses from bats—even though none of them had handled wildlife or reported SARS-like or other pneumonialike symptoms. Only one had traveled outside of Yunnan prior to the sampling, and all said they had seen bats flying in their village.

Three years earlier Shi's team had been called in to investigate the virus profile of a mine shaft in Yunnan's mountainous Mojiang County—famous for its fermented Pu'er tea—where six miners suffered from pneumonialike diseases and two died. After sampling the cave for a year, the researchers discovered a diverse group of coronaviruses in six bat species. In many cases, multiple viral strains had infected a single animal, turning it into a flying factory for new viruses.

"The mine shaft stunk like hell," says Shi, who, like her colleagues, went in wearing a protective mask and clothing. "Bat guano, covered in fungus, littered the cave." Although the fungus turned out to be the pathogen that had sickened the miners, she says it would have been only a matter of time before they caught the coronaviruses if the mine had not been promptly shut.

With growing human populations increasingly encroaching on wildlife habitats, with unprecedented changes in land use, with wildlife and livestock transported across countries and their products around the world, and with sharp increases in both domestic and international travel, pandemics of new diseases are a mathematical near certainty. This had been keeping Shi and many other researchers awake at night long before the mysterious samples landed at the Wuhan Institute of Virology on that ominous evening last December.

More than a year ago Shi's team published two comprehensive reviews about coronaviruses in *Viruses* and *Nature Reviews*

Microbiology. Drawing evidence from her own studies—many of which were published in top academic journals—and from others, Shi and her co-authors warned of the risk of future outbreaks of bat-borne coronaviruses.

Nightmare Scenario

On the train back to Wuhan on December 30 last year, Shi and her colleagues discussed ways to immediately start testing the patients' samples. In the following weeks—the most intense and the most stressful time of her life—China's bat woman felt she was fighting a battle in her worst nightmare, even though it was one she had been preparing for over the past 16 years. Using a technique called polymerase chain reaction, which can detect a virus by amplifying its genetic material, the team found that samples from five of seven patients had genetic sequences present in all coronaviruses.

Shi instructed her group to repeat the tests and, at the same time, sent the samples to another facility to sequence the full viral genomes. Meanwhile she frantically went through her own lab's records from the past few years to check for any mishandling of experimental materials, especially during disposal. Shi breathed a sigh of relief when the results came back: none of the sequences matched those of the viruses her team had sampled from bat caves. "That really took a load off my mind," she says. "I had not slept a wink for days."

By January 7 the Wuhan team had determined that the new virus had indeed caused the disease those patients suffered—a conclusion based on results from analyses using polymerase chain reaction, full genome sequencing, antibody tests of blood samples and the virus's ability to infect human lung cells in a petri dish. The genomic sequence of the virus, eventually named SARS-CoV-2, was 96 percent identical to that of a coronavirus the researchers had identified in horseshoe bats in Yunnan. Their results appeared in a paper published online on February 3 in *Nature*. "It's crystal clear that bats, once again, are the natural reservoir," says Daszak, who was not involved in the study.

Since then, researchers have published more than 4,500 genomic sequences of the virus, showing that samples around the world appear to "share a common ancestor," Baric says. The data also point to a single introduction into humans followed by sustained human-to-human transmission, researchers say.

Given that the virus seems fairly stable initially and that many infected individuals appear to have mild symptoms, scientists suspect that the pathogen might have been around for weeks or even months before severe cases raised the alarm. "There might have been mini outbreaks, but the viruses either burned out or maintained low-level transmission before causing havoc," Baric says. Most animal-borne viruses reemerge periodically, he adds, so "the Wuhan outbreak is by no means incidental."

Market Forces

To many, the region's burgeoning wildlife markets–which sell a wide range of animals such as bats, civets, pangolins, badgers and crocodiles–are perfect viral melting pots. Although humans could have caught the deadly virus from bats directly (according to several studies, including those by Shi and her colleagues), independent teams have suggested that pangolins may have been an intermediate host. These teams have reportedly uncovered SARS-CoV-2-like coronaviruses in pangolins that were seized in antismuggling operations in southern China.

On February 24 China announced a permanent ban on wildlife consumption and trade except for research, medicinal or display purposes–which will stamp out an industry worth $76 billion and put approximately 14 million people out of jobs, according to a 2017 report commissioned by the Chinese Academy of Engineering. Some welcome the initiative, whereas others, such as Daszak, worry that without efforts to change people's traditional beliefs or to provide alternative livelihoods, a blanket ban may simply push the business underground. This could make disease detection even more challenging. "Eating wildlife has been part of the cultural tradition" in China for thousands of years, Daszak says. "It won't change overnight."

In any case, Shi says, "wildlife trade and consumption are only part of problem." In late 2016 pigs across four farms in Qingyuan County in Guangdong–60 miles from the site where the SARS outbreak originated–suffered from acute vomiting and diarrhea, and nearly 25,000 of the animals died. Local veterinarians could not detect any known pathogen and called Shi for help. The cause of the illness–swine acute diarrhea syndrome (SADS)–turned out to be a virus whose genomic sequence was 98 percent identical to that of a coronavirus found in horseshoe bats in a nearby cave.

"This is a serious cause for concern," says Gregory Gray, an infectious disease epidemiologist at Duke University. Pigs and humans have very similar immune systems, making it easy for viruses to cross between the two species. Moreover, a team at Zhejiang University in the Chinese city of Hangzhou found that the SADS virus could infect cells from many organisms in a petri dish, including rodents, chickens, nonhuman primates and humans. Given the scale of swine farming in many countries, such as China and the U.S., Gray says, looking for novel coronaviruses in pigs should be a top priority.

The current outbreak follows several others during the past three decades that have been caused by six different bat-borne viruses: Hendra, Nipah, Marburg, SARS-CoV, MERS-CoV (Middle East respiratory syndrome) and Ebola. But "the animals [themselves] are not the problem," Wang says. In fact, bats promote biodiversity and ecosystem health by eating insects and pollinating plants. "The problem arises when we get in contact with them," he says.

Toward Prevention

When I spoke to Shi in late February–two months into the epidemic and one month after the government imposed severe movement restrictions in Wuhan, a megacity of 11 million–she said, laughing, that life felt almost normal. "Maybe we are getting used to it. The worst days are certainly over." The institute staffers had a special pass to travel from home to their lab, but they could not go anywhere else. They had to subsist on instant noodles during their long hours at work because the institute's canteen was closed.

New revelations about the coronavirus kept coming to light. The researchers discovered, for instance, that the pathogen enters human lung cells by using a receptor called angiotensin-converting enzyme 2, and they and other groups have since been screening for drugs that can block it. Scientists are also racing to develop vaccines. In the long run, the Wuhan team plans to develop broad-spectrum vaccines and drugs against coronaviruses deemed risky to humans. "The Wuhan outbreak is a wake-up call," Shi says.

Many scientists say the world should move beyond merely responding to deadly pathogens when they arise. "The best way forward is prevention," Daszak says. Because 70 percent of emerging infectious diseases of animal origins come from wildlife, a top priority should be identifying them and developing better diagnostic tests, he adds. Doing so would essentially mean continuing on a much larger scale what researchers such as Daszak and Shi had been doing before their funding ended this year.

Such efforts should focus on high-risk viral groups in mammals prone to coronavirus infections, such as bats, rodents, badgers, civets, pangolins and nonhuman primates, Daszak says. He adds that developing countries in the tropics, where wildlife diversity is greatest, should be the front line of this battle against viruses.

Daszak and his colleagues have analyzed approximately 500 human infectious diseases from the past century. They found that the emergence of new pathogens tends to happen in places where a dense population has been changing the landscape—by building roads and mines, cutting down forests and intensifying agriculture. "China is not the only hotspot," he says, noting that other major emerging economies, such as India, Nigeria and Brazil, are also at great risk.

Once potential pathogens are mapped out, scientists and public health officials can regularly check for possible infections by analyzing blood and swab samples from livestock, from wild animals that are farmed and traded, and from high-risk human populations such as farmers, miners, villagers who live near bats, and people who hunt or handle wildlife, Gray says. This approach, known as "One Health," aims to integrate the health management of wildlife, livestock and people. "Only then can we catch an outbreak before it turns into an epidemic," he says, adding that the strategy could potentially save the hundreds of billions of dollars such an epidemic can cost.

Back in Wuhan, where the lockdown was finally lifted on April 8, China's bat woman is not in a celebratory mood. She is distressed because stories from the Internet and major media have repeated a tenuous suggestion that SARS-CoV-2 accidentally leaked from her lab—despite the fact that its genetic sequence does not match any her lab had previously studied. Other scientists are quick to dismiss the allegation. "Shi leads a world-class lab of the highest standards," Daszak says.

Despite the disturbance, Shi is determined to continue her work. "The mission must go on," she says. "What we have uncovered is just the tip of an iceberg." She is planning to lead a national project to systematically sample viruses in bat caves, with much wider scope and intensity than previous attempts. Daszak's team has estimated that there are more than 5,000 coronavirus strains waiting to be discovered in bats globally.

"Bat-borne coronaviruses will cause more outbreaks," Shi says with a tone of brooding certainty. "We must find them before they find us."

About the Author

Jane Qiu is an award-winning science writer based in Beijing.

A High-Speed Scientific Hive Mind Emerged from the COVID Pandemic

By Joseph Bak-Coleman and Carl T. Bergstrom

Most of the time science is a slow and tedious business. Researchers toil away for decades at obscure limits of human knowledge, collecting and analyzing data, refining theories, writing, debating, and advancing our understanding of the world in tiny increments. Working in small teams on highly specialized projects far from the public eye—that is what most of us are accustomed to doing.

But a calamity upends everything. In early 2020, COVID spread around the globe. Millions of lives were at stake. Yet we knew next to nothing about the nature of the threat. Just a few months earlier no one had ever seen the SARS-CoV-2 virus.

For researchers, the emergence of the disease was an all-hands-on-deck moment. Biologists such as the two of us, along with virologists and immunologists, all pivoted to focus on the new pathogen. And other researchers from across the scientific ecosystem—economists, physicists, engineers, statisticians, psychologists, sociologists, and more—dropped everything to learn about COVID and figure out how they could contribute. Public interest exploded. Scientists with scant experience in public communication learned to work closely with journalists, informing a worried public about what was happening, what to expect next and what people could do to keep themselves safe. The scale of cooperation and collaboration is staggering. Large-scale surveys of scientists done in 2020 and 2021 show that roughly a third of researchers in the U.S. and Europe contributed to the effort.

This vast collaboration moved quickly and effectively in several areas. On December 30, 2019, an epidemiological surveillance network published the first English-language note about a cluster of pneumonia cases of unknown cause in Wuhan, China. Eight days later Chinese scientists identified the pathogen as a novel coronavirus. The full genome sequence was published just two days after that. Then on January 13, 2020, the World Health Organization published instructions for a PCR-based diagnostic test based on that genome.

The genome sequence also opened the door for vaccine development. Scientists used it to determine the 3-D structure of the SARS-CoV-2 spike protein, and by the end of January they had figured out how to stabilize the protein to make it an effective vaccine component, leading to mRNA-based and other vaccines, which were developed, tested and distributed in less than a year.

The urgency of COVID drove scientists to adapt. Discussions that previously took place at conferences, on the telephone or in revision notes on manuscripts moved to social media platforms such as Twitter, review sites such as PubPeer and all-hours Zoom rooms. Researchers and clinicians spontaneously organized into focused teams and working groups. By rapidly sharing information on their patients, physicians figured out that people with severe COVID were at high risk for dangerous blood clots in their lungs, so anticoagulants became a standard of care and saved lives.

In general, traditional modes of publication were far too slow. We embraced a rapid alternative model: preprint archives, where papers are posted prior to peer review or consideration at a scientific journal. The number of papers submitted to medRxiv, a key repository of biomedical preprints, increased 10-fold in the first few months of the pandemic.

These changes also shifted early-stage science from a private activity to part of the public discourse. Instead of presenting the world with polished scientific articles, investigators worked in open view, thinking aloud, offering preliminary speculations, arguing, making wrong turns, following dead ends and pursuing some hypotheses that would ultimately be refuted.

This approach to communication does have a downside. Previously private communications were now open to exploitation and distortion by politicians and pundits. For instance, flawed blood-sample research reported in an April 2020 medRxiv paper purported to show that COVID was a mild disease with a very low fatality rate. Although the scientific community quickly pointed out a host of problems with the work, people seeking to avoid business restrictions, school closures and mask mandates ignored the criticism and used the paper to undermine public health interventions.

Rapid and unorthodox channels of communication also could not solve all the problems scientists encountered. We took too long to recognize the importance of airborne transmission of the virus. We spent early 2020 washing our groceries but not wearing masks. Most critically, we have been largely unsuccessful at anticipating and managing the human element of the pandemic. By not accounting for ways that behavior would change in response to information—and misinformation—we have struggled to predict the size and timing of successive disease waves and virus variants. A collective failure to stop misinformation from spreading on social and traditional media platforms has left large segments of the population unvaccinated, vulnerable and unwilling to embrace measures such as masks and social distancing.

By some measures COVID has also hampered scientific productivity overall, researchers suggested in a paper in *Nature Communications* late last year. Some of the 2020 survey data revealed that scientists were spending an average of seven fewer hours per week working on research. The group, led by Dashun Wang of Northwestern University, wrote that the decrease in productivity will likely have lasting effects, with scientists reporting fewer publications, collaborations, submitted papers and new projects started during the pandemic. Lockdowns, school closures and other changes took a disproportionate toll on women scientists juggling work and child care—a major problem that requires urgent redress.

But a publication dip is precisely what we would expect when scientists shift from day-to-day research to an emergency response. Placing papers in journals becomes secondary to fixing problems. Dealing with urgent issues is one of the most important roles of the publicly funded scientific ecosystem, which has millions of researchers effectively on retainer. When global crises arise, they organize, learn and coordinate. And that, ultimately, leads to solutions.

About the Authors

Joseph Bak-Coleman is a postdoctoral fellow at the University of Washington Center for an Informed Public. He studies how communications technology affects collective decision-making.

Carl T. Bergstrom is a professor of biology at the University of Washington. He is a co-author of the report Science Education in the Age of Misinformation, *available online at sciedandmisinfo.stanford.edu.*

An mRNA Pioneer Discusses How Her Work Led to the COVID Vaccines

By Tanya Lewis

Researchers often toil away for years in a lab without any promise that their research will result in anything meaningful for society. But sometimes this work results in a breakthrough with global ramifications. Such was the case for Katalin Karikó, who, along with her colleague Drew Weissman, helped develop the messenger RNA (mRNA) technology that was used to produce the highly effective COVID vaccines made by Pfizer and Moderna.

Karikó, who is now senior vice president and head of RNA protein replacement therapies at BioNTech (the company that co-developed a COVID vaccine with Pfizer), and Weissman, a professor of vaccine research at the University of Pennsylvania's Perelman School of Medicine, have been awarded a $3 million Breakthrough Prize in Life Sciences for their work on modifying the genetic molecule RNA to avoid triggering a harmful immune response. The Breakthrough Prizes, founded by Sergey Brin, Priscilla Chan, Mark Zuckerberg, Yuri and Julia Milner, and Anne Wojcicki, honor groundbreaking discoveries in fundamental physics, life sciences and mathematics. (Earlier this year Karikó received the Vilcek Prize for Excellence in Biotechnology, a $100,000 award that recognizes the extraordinary contributions immigrants make to society and culture.) Karikó spent years on this research despite skepticism and a lack of funding. Ultimately, however, her efforts paid off—laying the groundwork for the overwhelmingly effective vaccines that are likely the world's surest way out of the COVID pandemic.

Karikó was born in Hungary to a family of modest means. She started her work on modifying RNA during her Ph.D. studies and—convinced of the promise of RNA-based therapies—came to the U.S. to pursue postdoctoral research. She later ended up as a professor at the University of Pennsylvania. Interest in mRNA therapies declined, and she was told to pursue other research directions or risk losing her position, but she persisted. Over a conversation at the Xerox machine she got to know Weissman, who was interested in developing vaccines at the time. They started collaborating.

When foreign mRNA is injected into the body, it causes a strong immune response. But Karikó and Weissman figured out a way to how to modify the RNA to make it less inflammatory by substituting one DNA "letter" molecule for another. Next they worked on how to deliver it. After testing many different delivery vehicles, they settled on lipid nanoparticles as the delivery vehicle. These turned out to work incredibly well: the nanoparticles acted as an adjuvant, a substance that enhances the desired immune response to a vaccine.

Weissman and his colleagues had been working on an mRNA vaccine for influenza when word spread of a mysterious pathogen causing pneumonia in people in Wuhan, China, in late 2019. Weissman quickly realized this virus was a perfect candidate for an mRNA vaccine, and Pfizer-BioNTech and Moderna soon pivoted to work on one. The rest is history.

Scientific American spoke with Karikó about how she came to work on mRNA, why it was well suited for COVID vaccines and what other exciting medical applications it could have.

[An edited transcript of the interviews follows.]

What was your initial reaction to winning the prize? Were you surprised, or did you expect this?

KARIKÓ: No, I never expected any kind of prize. For many decades, I never got anything. I was very happy with doing the work. Getting a letter from a New York elderly home where they celebrated that, with the vaccine, nobody died when they got the infection–for me, those are the real prizes. I was aware of this Breakthrough Prize–it's very famous. But, you know, I never thought about any kind of prize. So it was a very, very pleasant surprise.

Did you ever expect this technology to have such a global impact, in terms of the COVID vaccines? Or was it just something you were working on at the right place and time for this pandemic?

KARIKÓ: I never wanted to actually develop a vaccine. I was making this modification in the RNA because I always wanted to develop it for therapies. And when, in 2000, we learned that adding messenger RNA (which I made) to human immune cells, they made inflammatory molecules–cytokines–I thought that I had to do something. I tried to make sure that when we are using it for a therapy–you know, such as treating a patient who has had a stroke–we don't add some extra inflammatory molecules. At the beginning, it was thought that the immune form of this RNA would be a good vaccine. In 2017 the first paper was published showing that the modification we discovered that makes the mRNA noninflammatory could lead to a good vaccine, and the Moderna and BioNTech-Pfizer vaccines both have this modification.

Here at BioNTech, I am in charge of the protein replacement program. We use modified mRNA for cancer treatment. And this is not a vaccine. This is mRNA coding for cytokines and injecting them into tumors to make the tumor "hot" so that immune cells will learn what to see and can eliminate metastatic tumors. We did not know that there would be a pandemic, but I was aware that this is a very good way to make a vaccine because, with my colleagues at the University of Pennsylvania, we had already used it not just for Zika virus but for influenza, HIV, herpes simplex–it was already demonstrated in animal studies that it is such an excellent vaccine.

So when the pandemic started, was it immediately clear to you that this could be a useful technology to develop COVID vaccines?

KARIKÓ: From 2018 we had worked with Pfizer to develop a vaccine for influenza. And we were already ready to start a clinical trial for that. But switching over to COVID, it was just a technical thing. And so it was already ready.

If the pandemic had happened 20 years ago, you would need to have, physically, in your hands, a piece of the virus. So that would be a big delay. But commercial gene synthesis started about 20 years ago. Now you can just order a gene. You order DNA, and then you insert it into a [typically circular molecule of DNA called a] plasmid, and then you make RNA. But making the nanoparticle to deliver the mRNA is kind of challenging.

The lipid nanoparticles were a key part of the technology to make it useful for vaccines, right?

KARIKÓ: In my view, yes. The lipid nanoparticle protects the mRNA outside the cell because, in the blood and everywhere, there are a lot of human enzymes that can degrade the RNA. Second, it helps it to enter because the cell will pick up the particle. And then it is in the endosome [a membrane-bound compartment] in the immune cells, and then this lipid nanoparticle helps escape from the endosome to the cytoplasm [the solution inside cells] so the protein can be made. It is a very smart particle.

Do you see this technology being useful for many other types of applications, such as the cancer treatment you mentioned earlier?

KARIKÓ: It is already. When we started here at BioNTech, injecting messenger RNA coding for cytokines, by that time, the human trial using mRNA for cancer vaccines had already been going on for years. Other program with the nucleoside-modified mRNA was already ongoing at other companies. For example, Moderna is producing antibodies for chikungunya virus. [In a collaboration with AstraZeneca] they already have a phase II trial [led by the latter company] injecting mRNA into the heart [that] codes for [a protein that] generates new blood vessels. And they are also running a clinical trial for wound healing. So the data were out there–you already saw these ongoing trials for mRNA therapy–and it was just people who are not in the field who were not aware. They thought, "Oh, this is the first use." No, there are many, many other applications.

Has all this new interest in mRNA changed this field? Do you think it will accelerate the development of mRNA vaccines for other diseases, such as influenza?

KARIKÓ: Yeah, if you read the *Wall Street Journal* article [interviewing] Albert Bourla, CEO of Pfizer, you know, he said that Pfizer will pursue mRNA vaccines for other diseases. They will treat autoimmune disease. We published this year, at BioNTech, that we use tolerization [exposing someone to an antigen, or substance that provokes an immune response, until they can tolerate it]. We use an animal model for multiple sclerosis, and we showed that you can use tolerization to treat an autoimmune disease if the mRNA codes for the autoantigen. Before, it was like CureVac, Moderna, BioNTech—these were smaller companies working with RNA. And now, all of the sudden, you can see that Sanofi is buying into other companies, Pfizer is doing it, and so the large companies are realizing that they can get many products in their pipeline very quickly.

Do you think that this mRNA technology could be a good candidate for a universal coronavirus vaccine?

KARIKÓ: I think that it could work for all vaccines except those against bacterial infections. [It could work for vaccines against] viruses and parasites, such as [those that cause] malaria and, of course, for cancer—but we have to understand better what to target.

What do you plan to do with the prize money?

KARIKÓ: Probably, I will use it for research. I will make a company. When I got a smaller award, I gave it back to those who needed it more—for the education of underprivileged children. I am 66 years old and never had a new car, and I don't think I would have one now.

About the Author

Tanya Lewis is a senior editor covering health and medicine for Scientific American.

Messenger RNA Therapies Are Finally Fulfilling Their Promise

By Drew Weissman

In just 17 years, messenger RNA therapies went from proof of concept to global salvation. The Pfizer-BioNTech and Moderna vaccines for COVID-19 have been given to hundreds of millions of people, saving countless lives.

In 2005 Katalin Karikó and I created a way to make mRNA molecules that would not cause dangerous inflammation when injected into an animal's tissue. In 2017 Norbert Pardi and I demonstrated that modified mRNA, carried into human cells by a fatlike nanoparticle, was protected from being broken down by the body and prompted immune cells to generate antibodies that neutralize an invading virus more effectively than the immune system could on its own. The COVID vaccines made by Pfizer-BioNTech and Moderna both use this mRNA-liquid-nanoparticle "platform"–known as mRNA-LNP. In large clinical trials, it prevented more than 90 percent of the people who received the vaccines from becoming ill.

These extremely promising trials, and massive studies of people who have since received the vaccines, have finally given us sufficient information about the safety and efficacy of mRNA vaccines in humans. The platform outperformed more conventional approaches, in which vaccines are grown in laboratory cell cultures or chicken eggs. The rapid development also accelerated investment in further research. And because the U.S. Food and Drug Administration and similar regulatory agencies are now familiar with the technology, assessment of new therapeutics should come readily.

Messenger RNA vaccines instruct cells to create proteins that induce an immune response to an invader such as the SARS-CoV-2 virus, training the immune system to attack the actual pathogen if it infects the person in the future. These vaccines are easier to produce in large quantities than conventional protein therapies (genetically engineered versions of natural human or pathogen proteins) and monoclonal antibody therapies (lab-produced molecules that attack viruses in the same way that human antibodies do). And once a reliable manufacturing facility is built, it can quickly switch to a new mRNA vaccine or drug–unlike protein or monoclonal facilities, which must reengineer production from the ground up for each new therapy.

Success has inspired researchers, companies and government labs to pursue mRNA therapies for many infectious diseases, including influenza, cytomegalovirus, herpes simplex virus 2, norovirus, rabies, malaria, tuberculosis, dengue, Zika, HIV, hepatitis C and the entire family of coronaviruses. In each case, researchers wanted to determine exactly how mRNA-LNP vaccines induce potent antibody responses.

Work on mRNA vaccines also has expanded to certain cancers, food and environmental allergies, and autoimmune diseases. Positive results against ATTR amyloidosis, a fatal condition that involves the liver, have already been produced in a phase 1 clinical trial. Although the use of protein-based medications for certain illnesses is expanding quickly, large doses are typically required, and production is often difficult and expensive; mRNA delivery of therapeutic proteins could help. The approach has already worked in animals for issues as disparate as bone repair and asthma, and some treatments have advanced to human clinical trials. The Defense Advanced Research Projects Agency has even experimented with mRNA delivery of monoclonal antibodies that could be tailored for previously unidentified infectious diseases, with the goal of supplying reliable manufacturing of such remedies within 60 days.

The concentrated COVID work has also helped make mRNA a leader in nucleic acid therapeutics–approaches that can produce nearly any protein made by a specific cell. The technique is starting to be applied, and it could fight diseases in more convenient, less invasive and less expensive ways. For example, the fda has approved gene therapy for sickle cell anemia, and it is working in the U.S., although it requires marrow to be extracted from a person's bone, treated and reinserted; mRNA therapy could be delivered to marrow with a straightforward injection into a person's arm. If that works, sickle cell treatment could be greatly expanded in countries where the condition is widespread.

In a similar fashion, mRNA therapeutics could revolutionize the treatment of many infectious diseases in developing countries, greatly improving health-care equity. I have collaborated with labs around the world. Thai investigators at the vaccine center at Chulalongkorn in Bangkok and I made a Thai COVID vaccine and established a quality manufacturing center to produce it for Thailand and seven surrounding low- and middle-income countries. I undertook similar work in Africa and eastern Europe, with plans to extend it to South America.

Plenty of hurdles remain, including the creation of a better supply chain for delivering raw mRNA vaccine and materials needed for its production worldwide, as well as improvements that could reduce the dosage a person needs to receive. Yet the ease of mRNA production should enable most countries to make their own medications, as long as they can attract and retain researchers who can develop subsequent therapeutics that in turn keep domestic, high-quality manufacturing sites operating.

About the Author

Drew Weissman is a professor of vaccine research at the University of Pennsylvania. The nucleoside-modified mRNA-lipid-nanoparticle vaccine platform his laboratory created is used in COVID-19 vaccines made by Pfizer-BioNTech and Moderna. Weissman receives royalties from a patent for nucleoside-modified mRNA that is licensed by those two companies.

Pandemic-Era Research Will Pay Off for Years

By Britt Glaunsinger

After COVID appeared, a huge number of virologists, biochemists, cell biologists and immunologists shifted their work to the coronavirus, and because of that, the world got what it was desperately hoping for: a vaccine, in record time. Everything worked out better than we could have dreamed–several parallel vaccines, all with high efficacy. We are seeing antiviral treatments roll out, too.

Scientists can leverage all this effort to better understand other viruses and diseases. Never before have we been able to simultaneously test multiple vaccine platforms, head-to-head, in massive global clinical trials. Usually you are lucky if you get one vaccine to trial, and if it fails, you will not really know whether the concept or just the one platform failed.

I anticipate that scientists will use all the COVID research infrastructure to build more vaccines against other pathogens, such as cytomegalovirus and respiratory syncytial virus, and to create mRNA vaccines for flu. Furthermore, most of the coronavirus research has been collaborative. That will stick with people. It will make future work pay off more than if all those individuals went back to just their own niches.

This is not going to be the last spillover pandemic we see. It is not going to be the last public health crisis. I hope that COVID has given the public a sense of how important it is to have sustained investment in science. We don't know what discovery we will stumble on that will be the lifesaver the next time.

About the Author

Britt Glaunsinger is a molecular virologist at the University of California, Berkeley, and the Howard Hughes Medical Institute.

COVID Revealed the Fragility of American Public Health

By Wendy E. Parmet

Epidemics expose a society's vulnerabilities. And we were already an unhealthy population before COVID emerged. Compared with some other developed countries, the U.S. has extraordinary rates of chronic obstructive pulmonary disease, diabetes and other afflictions that leave people more susceptible to severe COVID. These vulnerabilities were influenced strongly by social factors–not purely genetics.

How did we get here? Partially it was because our public health system had been depleted and eroded. Public health has long been the second-class cousin of the individual health-care system, even though they are closely related. In recent history, we spent lots of money on individual treatment and invested far less in *population* health. Public health systems lacked adequate personnel, data systems for analysis, the latest technology and government support.

Adding to an already perilous situation, the pandemic exposed and accelerated preexisting trends in our society, such as growing distrust of institutions, including of science. In the past 20 years or more American conservatism transformed to antiscience populism. Even in the legal sphere, there has been a dramatic change in the past year in how many courts, including the U.S. Supreme Court, look at public health–a shift from perhaps being excessively deferential to public health policies to becoming hostile to public health, embracing an antiregulatory approach that spans various doctrinal categories.

With such a great push toward individualism, populism and a judicial review that is skeptical of public health, how do we keep the gains we've made against childhood diseases such as polio and measles, chronic illnesses such as those caused by smoking, and motor vehicle accidents? Life expectancy climbed in the 20th century not only because of tremendous scientific advancements and increasing wealth but also because public health campaigns and public health laws accomplished a lot. In the backlash against COVID restrictions and policy, we risk undoing all that.

About the Author

Wendy E. Parmet is faculty co-director of Northeastern University's Center for Health Policy and Law.

COVID Pushed Global Health Institutions to Their Limits

By Lawrence O. Gostin

Moments of existential crisis can turn into opportunities for bold reform. World War II led to the creation of transformative institutions–the United Nations in 1945 and the World Health Organization in 1948. The birth of the WHO came the same year that the U.N. adopted the Universal Declaration of Human Rights.

The COVID pandemic marks just such a moment of crisis. But instead of ushering in significant change, it has fractured global solidarity. That, in turn, has revealed deep-seated fragility in the WHO, the planet's health leader. The WHO's binding, governing framework for pandemic response–the International Health Regulations–has failed to serve its purpose in the face of widespread failures by national governments to comply.

But it is not too late to turn the corner. In fact, this is just the moment to ask what a bold new global public health architecture might look like.

As the U.N.'s first specialized agency, the WHO has a constitutional mandate to direct and coordinate international health, which includes advancing work to eradicate epidemic disease. No state acting alone can prevent the worldwide spread of infectious diseases. Only robust international institutions can set global norms, promote cooperation and share scientific information needed to respond to disease outbreaks. As a result, the WHO's role remains indispensable. With vast and growing global interdependency, intercontinental travel and mass migration, the realities of globalization and climate change have fueled a modern era of new diseases. The list includes three novel coronaviruses–SARS-CoV, MERS-CoV and SARS-CoV-2–and, of course, Ebola and Zika.

WHO director general Tedros Adhanom Ghebreyesus has been the world's conscience throughout the COVID crisis by urging global cooperation. But his pleas have largely been ignored by nationalistic leaders taking a stance of "my country first." Global dysfunction reached a pinnacle when President Donald Trump formally announced the U.S.'s intent to withdraw from the WHO. (President Joe Biden reversed this decision on his first day in office.) Yet Trump's was only one of many dysfunctional nationalistic responses, which ranged from near-total border closures to the hoarding by rich countries of personal protective equipment, oxygen and vaccines. The WHO was powerless to stop any of it. Even the agency's vaunted scientific expertise came into question, as it was embarrassingly late in recommending masks or acknowledging asymptomatic and aerosolized spread of the virus.

It is tempting to simply create an entirely new international health organization, but that would be a serious mistake. It took a world war to build political consensus to establish a global health agency with vast constitutional powers. Every country on Earth is a member except Liechtenstein and Taiwan (the latter left out because of the U.N.'s "One China" policy). The WHO helped to lead the efforts that brought about the eradication of smallpox and the near eradication of polio, among other crowning achievements. Instead of giving up on the agency, we should use this moment, and what political consensus we have, to prepare the organization for future pandemics—and what remains of the current one. This goal can be accomplished with robust funding and a bold new international agreement.

It has become painfully obvious that there is a major disconnect between what the world expects of the WHO and its capacities and powers. Consider its funding: The WHO's next Biennium Budget (for 2022 and 2023) is $6.12 billion, less than those of some large U.S. teaching hospitals and one fifth of the budget of the Centers for Disease Control and Prevention. As long ago as 2011, the WHO's report on the H1N1 influenza pandemic concluded that the agency's budget is "wholly incommensurate" with its global responsibilities. Yet the money it receives has remained roughly constant in inflation-adjusted dollars for the past three decades.

What is worse is that the WHO has control of less than 20 percent of its overall finances. That is the percentage of its budget that comes from so-called mandatory assessed contributions. The rest consists of voluntary contributions, which are mostly earmarked for donors' pet projects. The WHO cannot set global priorities or even hire for the long term, as voluntary funds disappear after a year. A donor then may just shift to another cause. Sustainable funding requires, at minimum, doubling the WHO's total budget over five years, with mandatory assessments making up at least 50 percent of its overall budget. Yet even these modest proposals might not pass muster, because member states insist on calling the shots as to how their contributions are used.

Beyond funding, the WHO must have enhanced powers to ensure governments work cooperatively in responding to global health emergencies. Yet the goal of enhancing the agency's powers involves several challenges. Most countries frowned on Trump's withdrawal from the WHO, but many agreed that he had a legitimate grievance. China's early reporting of COVID cases was disingenuous, causing a delay of weeks before the world was alerted, and the country later blocked an independent investigation of SARS-CoV-2's proximal origins. But what national leaders did not realize is that the WHO has no power to verify a nation's reports or gain entry to a state's territory for scientific investigations. These two structural weaknesses–and many more–are the subject of intense global negotiations to create a bold new pandemic treaty, perhaps taking advantage of the WHO's power to adopt broad-based, legally defined commitments such as the Framework Convention on Tobacco Control.

With crisis comes opportunity, and the new pandemic treaty has the potential to be transformative. It should introduce momentous reforms even beyond giving the WHO power to conduct independent investigations. These provisions should include adopting a "One Health" strategy (a collaborative and transdisciplinary approach to achieving optimal health outcomes) that recognizes the interconnection among people, animals, plants and their shared environments. The most likely origin of SARS-CoV-2 is a natural zoonotic spillover, the source of more than 60 percent of emerging diseases. Separating animal and human populations could prevent spillovers—a step that could be achieved through land management, reforestation and regulation of wild animal trade and markets.

Although SARS-CoV-2 most likely reached humans through natural means, a laboratory leak at the Wuhan Institute of Virology has been posed as an alternative theory for COVID's origins. Rigorous regulation and inspection of lab safety, as well as gain-of-function research, could help prevent the unintentional or deliberate release of novel pathogens.

Undoubtedly the rapid development of vaccines and therapeutics, including innovative messenger RNA technologies, was the greatest technological success in responding to the pandemic. But open access and sharing of data and tools, such as real-time virus samples, genomic sequencing, and results from clinical trials and other research, were often lacking. A new legal instrument negotiated under the auspices of the WHO's constitution could provide a pipeline for channeling significant research funding to where it is needed while promoting public-private partnerships and scientific cooperation.

Perhaps most important, the COVID pandemic revealed massive divides based on race, ethnicity, sex, disability and socioeconomic status at both international and national levels. High-income countries dominated global markets in diagnostics, protective equipment, therapeutics and, especially, vaccines. The WHO and its partners designed the Access to COVID-19 Tools (ACT) Accelerator to hasten the development and production of, and equitable access to, COVID resources. Yet COVAX (the ACT Accelerator's vaccine pillar) has badly underperformed. About 10 percent of Africa was fully vaccinated as of mid-January, compared with roughly 63 percent of the U.S. (the European Union had achieved even better coverage). COVAX could be transformative if it were properly funded and resourced and if its distribution channels were strengthened so that vaccines could be stored, transported and administered with speed and without waste.

President Biden has announced the investment of billions of dollars to expand mRNA-vaccine manufacturing, aiming for 100 million doses a month for domestic and global use. Yet this charitable-donation model is deeply flawed because donations always seem to come too little, too late. Any new international agreement must go beyond donations to plan for adequate and equitably distributed supplies of medical resources, including by securing supply chains, intellectual-property waivers, knowledge sharing and technology transfers.

I have delved into remaking global institutions, but it is obvious that we also must consider domestic public health capacities. The Global Health Security Index ranked the U.S. as most prepared for a pandemic, but the country was among the world's worst performers. There are many reasons for this lack of success, including a collapse of public trust and deep political polarization. But the CDC's guidance and actions–as well as those of state, local and tribal health departments–were, by any measure, weak. That agency and health departments at both state and local levels have lost considerable capacities (surveillance, labs and response) since the post-9/11 anthrax attacks. Buttressing domestic health system capacities is vital. But the CDC also erred badly in its health communications on topics ranging from asymptomatic and aerosolized spread to guidance on masks, vaccines and isolation. Its vaccine and mask recommendations, for example, changed three times in a matter of six weeks.

We are at a crucial junction in the COVID pandemic. We could simply return to the unvirtuous cycle of panic to neglect and back again. All too often, rather than building resilience during the pandemic response, we have blamed "the other," engaging in stereotyping of racial minorities and immersing ourselves in geostrategic battles. But we could transform this crisis into a historic opportunity for once-in-a-lifetime reforms of our national and global health systems based on science, equity and solidarity.

About the Author

Lawrence O. Gostin is University Professor (Georgetown University's highest academic rank) and Founding O'Neill Chair in Global Health Law and a professor of medicine at Georgetown. He is also director of the World Health Organization Collaborating Center for National and Global Health Law.

Section 3: How COVID-19 Changed Society

3.1 COVID Has Made Global Inequality Much Worse
By Joseph E. Stiglitz

3.2 COVID Has Created a Perfect Storm for Fringe Science
By David Robert Grimes

3.3 COVID Changed the World of Work Forever
By Christina Maslach and Michael P. Leiter

3.4 How a Virus Exposed the Myth of Rugged Individualism
By Robin G. Nelson

3.5 How the Pandemic Remade Science Journalism
By Tanya Lewis

3.6 Introducing 21 Ways COVID Changed the World
By Jen Schwartz

COVID Has Made Global Inequality Much Worse

By Joseph E. Stiglitz

The novel coronavirus exposed and exacerbated the fragility and inequity of the global economic system. Many countries, including the U.S., proved unable to manufacture simple products such as face masks, let alone more complicated ones such as ventilators. Multiple supply chains broke. The resulting ordeal will almost surely lead to the creation of more onshore production facilities. An ugly nationalism displayed by countries that have hoarded vaccines and put profits over lives shows no sign of abating, despite its potentially devastating outcomes for the world.

The pandemic's most significant outcome will be a worsening of inequality, both within the U.S. and between developed and developing countries. Global billionaire wealth grew by $4.4 trillion between 2020 and 2021, and at the same time more than 100 million people fell below the poverty line. Just how bad the situation will become depends on how long the disease rages and what policy makers do to control it and its consequences.

In part because of its huge income and wealth inequalities, the U.S. suffered the most COVID-attributed deaths of any country. SARS-CoV-2 went after those with poverty-related health conditions and with jobs that cannot be done in isolation. Surviving from paycheck to paycheck and not having even the most basic rights of health care and paid sick leave, many Americans lacked testing to know if they were infected and either went to work, spreading the virus, or sought help too late.

The poorest will also suffer the most from the pandemic's economic aftermath–in particular, from the loss of jobs, disproportionately concentrated in low-wage service sectors. Just as worrisome, poorer children have experienced terrible educational setbacks as schools moved online, presaging a potentially long-term aggravation of inequality and deprivation.

Still, a strong policy response in the U.S. has created a shallower economic downturn than elsewhere. President Joe Biden's American Rescue Plan *reduced* childhood poverty in 2021 by more than a third, demonstrating that the country's high level of poverty has always been a matter of choice. But the measures taken so far are temporary palliatives. The Build Back Better plan was designed to make these achievements more permanent and to reduce inequality in all its dimensions. If it fails to pass, we can expect an enduring increase in poverty. Matters will almost surely get even worse if the pandemic continues.

It was a triumph of scientific, political and economic organization that we were able to so quickly develop, produce and distribute billions of vaccine doses. But matching these enormous successes are colossal failures. Despite having the technology and the resources, we have failed to ramp up vaccine supply and distribute enough doses in poor countries.

Markets can solve most economic problems—a shortage of glass vials, for example. They cannot, however, overcome the legal barriers presented by intellectual-property rights that have given the current producers of vaccines monopoly power. Those pharmaceutical companies have an incentive to restrict manufacturing, allowing them to charge prices that are a multiple of the cost of production—although most of the original R&D, and even much of the initial productive capacity, was publicly financed.

The failure to bring the disease under control and the unequal burden of the disease are thus largely a failure of our economic and political systems. Had a vaccine intellectual-property waiver, which would allow any firm in the world to produce the vaccines after paying a fair royalty, been adopted when it was first proposed in 2020, we would almost surely have far greater supplies today. Hope may have arrived in the form of CORBEVAX, a vaccine that has no patent restrictions and is easy to make, circumventing national selfishness and corporate greed. If it proves sufficiently safe and effective, it could get the world inoculated, reducing the likelihood of a more deadly, more contagious or vaccine-resistant mutation.

The global inequities in vaccine distribution are matched by glaring inequities in responses to the economic downturn. Whereas the U.S. spent a quarter of its gross domestic product (GDP) to keep the economy going, poor countries could spend but a mere fraction of that amount. Some countries have seen a drop in GDP of 10 percent or more, with especially adverse effects on the poorest. And although the U.S. can manage the large increase in debt, poor nations will find it difficult to do so.

Unfortunately, then, the economic shock of the pandemic most likely will linger. It will be those at the bottom—poorer Americans and most people in poorer countries—who will still suffer the consequences years from now. Not doing everything we can to control the disease and its economic aftermath *everywhere* is shortsighted. Dithering and dawdling will allow COVID to rage on, with further supply chain disruptions contributing to shortages, postponing a robust global recovery and entrenching unconscionable levels of inequality.

About the Author

Joseph E. Stiglitz is a University Professor at Columbia University and chief economist at the Roosevelt Institute. He received the Nobel prize in economics in 2001. Stiglitz chaired President Bill Clinton's Council of Economic Advisers from 1995 to 1997 and served as the chief economist and senior vice president of the World Bank from 1997 to 2000. He chaired the Sarkozy commission (2008–2009) and an expert group (2013–2019) at the OECD for devising measures for well-being and sustainability.

COVID Has Created a Perfect Storm for Fringe Science

By David Robert Grimes

The explosion of disinformation about COVID has been a defining aspect of the pandemic. Alongside the virus itself, we've been shadowed by what the World Health Organization has called an infodemic. This is widely known, of course, but much less discussed is the role of ostensible "experts" in perpetuating dangerous fictions. Since the dawn of the crisis, a disconcerting number of eminently qualified scientists and physicians have propagated falsehoods across social media, elevating themselves to the status of gurus in order to lend a veneer of seeming scientific legitimacy to empty, dangerous claims. And these bogus claims, like their pathological namesake, have gone uncontrollably viral.

In March 2020, for example, physician Thomas Cowan insisted that COVID-19 was caused by 5G radio frequencies. Although this assertion was both devoid of evidence and physically impossible, this proved no impediment to widespread acceptance, with anti-5G sentiment accounting for at least 87 arson attacks on cell-phone towers in the U.K. alone. The ostensible documentary *Plandemic*, starring Ph.D. virologist Judy Mikovits, ratcheted up millions of views with the central thesis that coronavirus is a planned hoax. Even Nobel laurates in medicine have been culpable; Luc Montagnier's statement that COVID was likely manufactured earned him both the enthusiastic embrace of conspiracy theorists and the enmity of scientific peers who refuted the conjecture as utterly false.

Ineffective treatments ranging from hydrochloroquine to ivermectin to vitamin D and alternative medicine have thrived too, endorsed by a rogues' gallery of doctors and researchers. Even now, as the life-saving impact of vaccination begins to be felt across the globe, a new cohort of impressively credentialed contrarians has emerged, spreading mistruths about immunization. The grandiosely named

"World Doctors Alliance" is a potent example, boasting amongst its membership physician Vernon Coleman (an anti-vaccine activist and author of a book insisting COVID is a hoax) and Dolores Cahill, the once-respected Irish scientist whose conspiratorial proclamations have become a staple of lockdown protests and COVID denialist disinformation across Europe.

In slickly produced videos shared relentlessly online, these fringe scientists are lauded as experts unafraid to speak truth to power. But it is crucial to note that these individuals, for all their formal credentials, extol a narrative completely at odds with reality, readily refuted by public health bodies the world over. These pseudoscientific, conspiratorial claims are archetypal arguments from authority, where a perceived expert's support is used to justify positions unsupported by data. Scientific claims do not derive their authority by virtue of coming from scientists, but from the weight of the evidence behind them. Pseudoscience, by contrast, tends to focus on ostensible gurus rather than consensus opinion. The only authority a scientist can ever truly invoke is a reflected one, dependent on accurately representing the evidence base. If they embrace fringe positions and jettison the principles of scientific skepticism, then their qualifications, education and prestige mean absolutely nothing.

Were these claims merely vapid that would be bad enough. Yet they are also uniquely damaging to public understanding. Scientists and physicians occupy an extremely trusted position in society, and an imprimatur of scientific legitimacy is a powerful one. This is a trust utterly abused by fringe figures, who present qualifications as a proxy for scientific validity. This is superficially convincing to the point that it does not matter that these videos originated in conspiratorial circles; the intrinsic aura of "science" afforded by apparent experts enables them to metastasize far beyond this odious origin. This in turn casts a specter of doubt over the advice of public health bodies, distorting public understanding by presenting rank fictions in the stolen robes of science.

The rise of pseudoexperts is perhaps symptomatic of a change in how we access information. As we become curators of our own media, the traditional gatekeepers and fact-checkers once implicit in most reporting have been increasingly sidelined. This in turn has made us more polarized, and reduced our ability to differentiate fact from opinion. Motivated reasoning, our human bias towards cherry-picking only arguments that chime with that we wish were true, most certainly plays a role. The impositions of COVID are manifold; it is not surprising that fringe scientists are inevitably invoked as sources for those with strong feelings against lockdowns, masks and vaccination. Even if we are not ideologically predisposed to such positions, these claims undermine public understanding, blurring perceptions of scientific consensus, nudging us collectively towards fear and distrust.

The dark irony is that these fringe figures weaponize the societal trust afforded to science, unduly amplifying their capacity to unleash serious harm. To mitigate this, we need to keep in mind the vital distinction "science" and "scientists." Individual scientists are far from infallible; they can be fooled by subtle mistakes, haunted by spurious conclusions or even become so ideologically wedded to a belief they bend facts to fit that preconception. Their motivations are human; they can be seduced by the lure of money, infamy or admiration. Science, by contrast, is a systemic method of inquiry, where positions are formed on the totality of evidence. Crucially, to be labeled "scientific," ideas should be testable, and those that fail to withstand dispassionate investigation are duly discarded.

For all their qualifications, fringe scientists fail this basic tenet of science, as they are united in their willingness to embrace conspiracy theory when their claims are refuted. Lack of evidence for their position is airily dismissed as a cover-up by everyone from the WHO to the entire medical establishment. But this performative outrage is so much sound and fury to distract from the inescapable reality that their positions are completely contradicted by the overwhelming weight of scientific evidence. This is scientifically reprehensible, and staggeringly irresponsible, conduct.

It is entirely understandable that many are left confused and uneasy by the vocal assertions of fringe figures, but the onus of proof is always on those making grand claims. The history of science and medicine is littered with the hubris of the arrogant and misguided, and mere credentials are no impediment to being wrong; only evidence truly matters. When confronted with the pronouncement of fringe figures, the motto of the Royal Society should always be at for forefront of our mind: "*Nullius in verba*" (take nobody's word for it).

About the Author

David Robert Grimes is a scientist and author of Good Thinking: Why Flawed Logic Puts Us All at Risk and How Critical Thinking Can Save the World *(The Experiment, 2021). His work focuses on health disinformation and conspiracy theory, and he is an international advocate for the public understanding of science. Grimes is a recipient of the Nature/Sense about Science Maddox Prize and a fellow of the Committee for Skeptical Inquiry.*

COVID Changed the World of Work Forever

By Christina Maslach and Michael P. Leiter

Hardly anyone has made it through the pandemic with their work life unchanged. Millions of people have lost jobs, been placed on furlough or switched to working from home. Essential workers have continued in place but often with major changes to their workloads, including additional safety procedures and an awareness of infectious disease as a new workplace hazard. According to the Bureau of Labor Statistics, employment dropped by 20.5 million people in the U.S. alone in April 2020. Service providers were hit most intensely: 7.7 million jobs were lost in the leisure and hospitality sector, with 5.5 million of them in food service or drinking establishments.

The shift to remote work led to the complete collapse of the work-home boundary, especially for parents juggling child care and homeschooling with job demands. Poorly timed or endless Zoom meetings interfered with people's ability to get work done and sometimes harmed relationships with colleagues. Essential workers often discovered that their employers' only strategy to bridge the gap created by increased demand was for them to work harder–reinforcements were not on the way. Many employees had to deal with inadequate personal protective equipment while feeling unfairly treated. And it became more difficult for everyone to relax and recover from their ongoing exhaustion as entertainment and fitness facilities closed. Because of these changes, workers experienced more stressful exhaustion, became more negative and cynical about the workplace and felt an erosion of self-confidence–the triple markers of burnout.

At the same time, other people–especially those with comfortable home offices and few parental responsibilities–found benefits in working remotely. Being on their own gave them greater control with fewer distractions. The absence of commuting gave people more time and energy while saving them money. People who had been working in unpleasant or hostile workplaces were now free from disrespectful encounters.

The pandemic has taught many people that the job does not have to be the way it was. This realization may be one reason that many are not going back to their old jobs. At the end of 2021, the service provider and hospitality sectors were facing major challenges in enticing people back to these low-paid, heavy-demand jobs, with many positions remaining empty. At the same time, 4.5 million Americans (3 percent of the workforce) voluntarily quit their jobs in November, reflecting both discontent with their current positions and the desire to fid better ones. But solving the burnout problem cannot fall to individual workers. The workplace must change. People burn out because their employers have not successfully managed chronic job stressors. We must place a stronger focus on modifying or redesigning workplace conditions. How can job environments be places that help people thrive rather than wearing them down?

People whose work lives got better over the past two years can generally thank personal resources–a comfortable room of one's own–rather than foresight from their employers. But employers can learn a lot from attending to what helped people be more productive and satisfied during this time. For example, workers were less distracted by pointless meetings and open office settings and were able to focus on meaningful tasks rather than being burdened by busywork. Some companies are trying to entice workers with higher pay or time off. Improving job conditions has even more potential for enduring impact.

Work takes up a lot of people's time, talent and potential–and workers are increasingly demanding that it offer a sustainable and rewarding quality of life in return.

About the Authors

Christina Maslach is a professor of psychology at the University of California, Berkeley, and creator of the Maslach Burnout Inventory, a widely used psychological instrument. She and Leiter co-authored The Burnout Challenge *(Harvard University Press, 2022).*

Michael P. Leiter is an organizational psychologist and president of Michael Leiter & Associates, a consulting firm in Nova Scotia.

How a Virus Exposed the Myth of Rugged Individualism

By Robin G. Nelson

For countless Americans, there was a dull but persistent pain to prepandemic life: high-priced housing, nearly inaccessible health care, underresourced schools, wage stagnation and systemic inequality. It was a familiar ache, a kind of chronic hurt that people learned to live with simply because they had no other choice. Faced with threadbare safety nets and a cultural ethos championing nationalist myths of self-sufficiency, many people did what humans have always done in times of need: they sought emotional comfort and material aid from their family and friends. But when COVID-19 hit, relying on our immediate networks was not sufficient. Americans are gaslit into thinking that they are immeasurably strong, impervious to the challenges people in other countries face. In reality, our social and economic support systems are weak, and many people are made vulnerable by nearly any change in their capacity to earn a living. The fallout from the pandemic is an urgent call to strengthen our aid systems.

Anthropologists have long recognized that exceptionally high degrees of sociality, cooperation and communal care are hallmarks of humankind, traits that separate us from our closest living relatives, the chimpanzees and bonobos. This interdependence has been key to our success as a species. Viewed this way, we humans have an evolutionary mandate to be generous and take care of one another. But unlike early humans, who lived in comparatively small groups, we cannot just rely on our immediate family and friends for support. We must invest in national policies of communal care—policies that facilitate access to resources for people who need help—to a degree that is commensurate with the size and complexity of today's globalized societies.

In a sense, the entanglement of our everyday lives made us all the more vulnerable to an airborne virus that demanded social isolation, blowing up the facade of normalcy in the spring of 2020. The new COVID normal, with its mask wearing, social distancing, lockdowns and closed schools, compelled us to abandon our most basic instincts and turn away from our closest friends and family. It rent the social fabric on which we all rely.

Infectious diseases present an unusual challenge: to combat them effectively, we must render aid appropriately and consistently at scale. This pandemic exposed the fragility and faults in each layer of our lives—from our innermost circle of family and friends to the nation state at the periphery—and the differential risk experienced by any individual's core community. Communities that were already heavily invested in social safety nets with measures such as paid sick leave were able to lower COVID rates. Those invested in the ideology of self-sufficiency and individualism prolonged suffering and loss of life.

New Zealand (Aotearoa in Māori), a country with a long history of reckoning with its colonial past and building community, has been a standout success story in the pandemic. The government there countered COVID with nationwide stay-at-home orders, border controls, hygiene campaigns, accessible testing and contact tracing. The results were dramatic: 18 months into the pandemic, the country had seen only 27 COVID deaths. By late 2021, 90 percent of eligible citizens were fully vaccinated. Although new variants have been challenging these successes, the government remains deeply committed to care.

Similarly, Taiwan defied predictions that it would struggle with COVID infections like its neighbors in China by instituting a 14-day isolation policy for travelers entering the country, stepping up mask production, increasing border controls and deputizing quarantine officers who could help isolated citizens. By March 2021 there had been only 10 COVID deaths in a country of nearly 24 million people. Taiwan has fought each new wave of the pandemic with these tactics. Although we may call on our inner circle most frequently during our times of need, ultimately we must rely on local and national officials on the periphery of our lives to be exquisitely human—as the leaders of New Zealand and Taiwan have been—when they develop and enact health policies.

In the U.S., government support was inconsistent, and citizens struggled to work together to keep the virus at bay. The roots of these problems run deep. Since this country's inception, the dominant ideologies here have encouraged not only individualism but also the dehumanization of certain groups, as evidenced by the enslavement of Black people and the displacement of Indigenous communities from their ancestral lands. This dehumanization continues today in the form of the bootstrap narrative—the myth that anyone can prosper if only they work hard enough—and in efforts to weaken relief programs for people who need help. As a result, even though we now know how the virus spreads and causes disease and we have effective vaccines against it, the death toll from COVID is higher in the U.S. than anywhere else.

There have been some success stories in the U.S.—they can be found in groups that have a fundamentally different ideological relationship to community interdependence. The Navajo Nation, which early on saw some of the highest rates of COVID-related illness and death, ran its own vaccine education campaigns and implemented in-house vaccine-distribution policies. It achieved far higher vaccination rates on its reservations than surrounding areas did. Tribal values that prioritize the group over the individual helped motivate members to get their shots. Unfortunately, in late 2021 the virus surged among the Navajo again, perhaps because of low vaccination rates in neighboring areas.

A microbe revealed the lie of rugged individualism. We are not self-sufficient and independent; we never have been. Our fates are bound together. Taking care of others is taking care of ourselves. With the arrival of the highly infectious Omicron variant, we are paying the price for not having developed strong policies early on and stuck to them. But that does not mean we should just give up the fight. Instead we need to redouble our efforts to provide care and resources to vulnerable community members. The emergence of each new COVID variant is an opportunity to reflect on what worked and what did not with the last one, whether locally or on the other side of the world. Committing ourselves to upholding our evolutionary mandate to help one another—not just the people we see every day but everyone, everywhere—is the only thing that will save us.

About the Author

Robin G. Nelson is a biological anthropologist at Arizona State University. She studies human sociality and health outcomes through the lens of evolutionary theory.

How the Pandemic Remade Science Journalism

By Tanya Lewis

When I first heard the reports of a "mysterious pneumonia" spreading in Wuhan, China, in January 2020, I thought I would write a story or two about it and move on to the next big medical news development. As a health journalist, disease outbreaks are not a rare occurrence on my beat, and most do not rise to the level of an international emergency. But the story of COVID-19 would turn out to be unlike anything I had covered before or am likely—I hope—to ever cover again.

Reporting on the pandemic was like building a plane while flying it—at warp speed in a hurricane. The underlying science was evolving daily, so there was no expert consensus or body of established research to draw on. And there were plenty of people willing to exploit this information vacuum, creating a secondary epidemic of misinformation.

Early on Chinese authorities suppressed information about the virus, and the Trump administration downplayed its threat to the U.S. Testing blunders and shortages prevented this country from recognizing the number of COVID cases circulating within its borders in the critical early phase when we could have slowed its spread. And for months health authorities said SARS-CoV-2 was spread primarily by symptomatic people through large respiratory droplets from a cough or a sneeze or by contaminated surfaces (remember the now ridiculous-seeming grocery-disinfecting ritual?). That guidance was based on how some other respiratory diseases circulate, but of course we now know this novel coronavirus commonly spreads through aerosols that linger in the air, often exhaled by a person showing no symptoms at all.

At the heart of science journalism is a focus on evidence. But one of the hardest lessons many other journalists and I learned while reporting on COVID is that absence of evidence is not evidence of absence–and that even advice from renowned public health authorities should sometimes be questioned. Take face masks, for example: in the pandemic's first crucial weeks, the Centers for Disease Control and Prevention and the World Health Organization said the public did not need to wear masks (despite the fact that medical workers and many people in Asia use them routinely to protect against respiratory diseases). At the same time, CDC and WHO officials specifically told people not to buy high-quality respirator masks because health-care workers needed them–breeding confusion and mistrust.

At the time, I debated with my editor over whether to recommend that people wear masks, against the guidance of these esteemed health agencies. I resisted doing so, in part out of deference to these authorities and in part because of a lack of published studies that masks–especially nonmedical ones–were protective for the wearer. In retrospect, I should have followed the precautionary principle; in the absence of direct evidence, masks were a reasonable precaution to protect against a respiratory virus. That episode highlighted for me just how challenging it can be when the evidence is shifting in real time and even the experts can't keep up. It wasn't until two years into the pandemic that the CDC and others finally started to emphasize the importance of high-filtration masks, which had been abundantly available in the U.S. for many months.

It didn't take long for bad actors to weaponize the confusion to spread misinformation. Patient zero in this "infodemic" was Donald Trump. The former president routinely downplayed the virus's severity, calling it "no worse than the flu." He blamed China, stoking xenophobia rather than urging people to protect themselves and others. He mocked people who wore masks, politicizing a basic public health measure, while promoting baseless COVID treatments. It wasn't just Trump–Fox News personalities and celebrities such as Joe Rogan and Aaron Rodgers have used their platforms to spread falsehoods about the virus and the vaccines. As a health journalist, my job was no longer purely about explaining the science–I now had to contend with politics and human behavior. Actions as seemingly innocuous as wearing a mask or getting a vaccine to avoid getting a disease had become political statements.

There has perhaps been no more consequential or bitter battleground in the U.S. epidemic than vaccines. The anti-vax movement—a small faction but already a potent force before COVID—took advantage of people's hesitancy about the speed with which the new vaccines were developed to spread lies and misinformation about their effects. COVID anti-vaxxers promoted their dangerous claims under the guise of "freedom," never acknowledging that it comes at the cost of people's lives and the freedom to live without threat of a deadly virus. As science journalists, it was not enough just to report the facts and debunk misinformation—we had to engage with the reasons people believe such falsehoods. We learned to use the latest research on how misinformation spreads to try to expose lies without amplifying them and replace conspiracy theories with truth.

All of this has played out against the backdrop of vast inequities in access to vaccines and health care, both nationwide and globally. One of the biggest lessons of the pandemic for many of us has been that racism, not race, explains why COVID has been even more devastating for people of color.

The arrival of new viral variants further complicated messaging. The mRNA vaccines achieved an effectiveness beyond any expert's wildest dreams. But their protection waned over time, and they have been less effective against the highly contagious Delta and Omicron variants, prompting a return to mask wearing and a hastily implemented booster shot campaign. As I write this, Omicron is spreading rapidly and overwhelming hospitals because it is so transmissible. As journalists, all we can do is try to make sense of the evidence as it develops, hope in hindsight we made the right call, and remind readers it's normal, not bad, to update our knowledge as the virus—and our understanding of it—evolves.

Reporting on COVID has fundamentally changed the way I approach science journalism. I have gained a deeper appreciation for scientific knowledge as a process, not merely an end result. I have seen that it is not enough to simply follow the science–that skepticism of authority is warranted even when that authority comes from respected public health experts. And I have learned that science is *always* political–despite what many scientists like to think. These lessons have been won at a terrible expense. But failing to heed them could doom us to repeat this tragedy when the next pandemic comes.

About the Author

Tanya Lewis is a senior health and medicine editor at Scientific American. *She co-hosts a biweekly podcast, COVID Quickly, with fellow senior medicine editor Josh Fischman.*

Introducing 21 Ways COVID Changed the World

By Jen Schwartz

In the spring of 2020 a cartoon was making the rounds on social media. It showed a city perched on a tiny island, surrounded by ocean. A speech bubble emerged from the skyline: "Be sure to wash your hands and all will be well." Not far out at sea, a giant wave labeled "COVID-19" was about to crash over the city. Behind it was an even bigger wave marked "recession." And beyond that one was a tower of water that threatened to swallow it all: "climate change."

I've often thought of that statement, by Canadian cartoonist Graeme MacKay, in moments that seem to define our pandemic disorientation: the botched messaging, willful unpreparedness and exhausted confusion. In America, though, the cartoon didn't play out exactly as drawn. The economy actually *grew* in 2021. Does that mean the damage wasn't as bad as many predicted? That question can only be answered in the context of another superlative: the U.S. claims the highest reported number of COVID cases–as well as COVID deaths–in the world.

The past two years have been full of incongruities, paradoxes and absurdities. Consider the mRNA vaccines. Scientists formed a global hive mind and delivered a supereffective vaccine faster than anyone thought possible. But more than a year after the shots became available, the U.S. has one of the lowest vaccination rates among wealthy countries. Some Americans think the vaccine represents a weapon of oppression, if not a literal weapon.

The politicization of our best tool for ending the pandemic surprised everyone. Except for the behavioral scientists, misinformation researchers, sociologists, historians and speculative fiction writers who spent 2020 waving their arms (sometimes in the pages of this magazine), calling attention to cognitive bias, influence operations, accessibility issues and barriers to trust.

COVID was never going to be the "common enemy" that finally united Americans. As Alondra Nelson, who is now deputy director for science and society at the White House Office of Science and Technology Policy, explained it to me in December 2020: "This idyllic idea of solidarity, especially in a wartime modality, is created by making an enemy of someone else." Indeed, former president Donald Trump tried to make an enemy by blaming the virus on China. His xenophobic rhetoric has spread, feeding dangerous conspiracy theories, threatening scientific research and leading to a rise in hate crimes.

The virus provoked other reckonings and pivots–not all of them bad. Many of us who could do our jobs remotely discovered the power of owning our time. COVID concerns made it easier for European cities to install miles and miles of bike lanes, giving us a glimpse of a car-free urban future. The pandemic revealed strange hidden interdependencies; hospital demand for liquid oxygen, for example, delayed rocket launches. It also worsened inequality, increased the prevalence of depressive disorders, added "moral injury" to the common lexicon and set back students' learning trajectories for years to come.

Amid the noise of an ongoing emergency, it can be hard to notice troubling new trends. We should be far more concerned about the shadow of long COVID. If millions of people end up developing persistent health issues after the acute disease stage, they will likely encounter a medical system unable to do much more than shrug. As with the climate crisis, many of us avert our eyes from the specter of long COVID because its effects tend to be more insidious than dramatic, and the fixes aren't quick or easy. Dealing with the problem requires acknowledging what was already broken. Yet for every bleak future there's a hopeful one. Propelled by the force of patient advocates, research into long COVID could lead to new understanding of other postinfection illnesses and autoimmune disorders.

When we planned this issue, Omicron had not yet emerged. I wondered if people would be interested in stories about a pandemic that wasn't over, even if they were over the pandemic. Would we be fearmongering to suggest that the pandemic hasn't ended because we haven't vaccinated the world, leaving us susceptible to variants that are more transmissible?

We're *all* over COVID. But we can't give up and leave our collective fate to the machinations of a virus, sighing in relief when one peak crests (for those of us still unharmed) and leaning on wishful thinking that only the best-case scenarios will come to pass. Avoiding adaptation isn't the key to reaching the endemic stage, nor will it help us prepare for the even bigger waves of climate crises. We assembled this collection of stories to reflect on how COVID has already changed our world, as well as how our world has been resistant to change—even when a virus disrupts everything, even when it shows us what we need to change the most.

About the Author

Jen Schwartz is a senior editor of features at Scientific American *who covers how people are adapting, or not, to a rapidly changing world.*

Section 4: Meanwhile, Other Epidemics

4.1 The Biggest Health Problem: Obesity
By Mercedes Carnethon

4.2 The Opioid Epidemic Is Surging among Black People because of Unequal Access to Treatment
By Melba Newsome and Gioncarlo Valentine

4.3 Doctors Need to Learn to Talk about Suicide
By Rodolfo Bonnin and Leonard M. Gralnik

4.4 Why Does Ebola Keep Showing Up in the Democratic Republic of the Congo?
By Dina Fine Maron

4.5 Ebola Outbreak in Uganda Surges, but the Country Has a Plan
By Paul Adepoju

4.6 "Their Lives Are Worth More Than Ours": Experts in Africa Slam Global Response to Monkeypox
By Paul Adepoju

4.7 We Can't Let Monkeypox Turn into a Repeat of COVID
By Muhammad Jawad Noon

The Biggest Health Problem: Obesity

By Mercedes Carnethon

As the chief of epidemiology at a major medical school, I am frequently asked what the biggest threat is to the health of our nation. My response is obesity.

The obesity epidemic is a public health crisis in the U.S. Over one-third of all adults are obese; and another two-thirds are overweight and on the way to becoming obese. In racial and ethnic minority groups including blacks, Hispanics and Native Americans, obesity has touched nearly half of the adult population.

That is why I cheered when I read the findings of a recent study describing how effective a beverage tax was on lowering the consumption of sugar-sweetened beverages in Philadelphia.

The logical first line of defense against obesity is individual behavior changes to promote healthy lifestyles. However, individual behavior change is ineffective in the face of social and structural barriers that constrain individual choice. These barriers are uniquely relevant among racial and ethnic minorities and impoverished adults who are more likely to be obese.

Across a lifetime, obesity contributes to the development of physical illnesses including cardiovascular diseases and lung disease, mental illnesses such as depression, and disabilities including osteoarthritis.

Obesity is also responsible for perpetuating disparities in multiple chronic diseases by race, ethnicity and socioeconomic class. For example, the disparate burden of obesity in blacks may explain elevated rates of heart failure and stroke in black men and women as compared with whites.

One reason why I support using sin taxes such as the sugared beverage tax to regulate unhealthy behaviors that contribute to obesity is because their reach is broader than individual interventions.

The "prevention paradox" as described by British epidemiologist Geoffrey Rose in a 1985 study that was republished in 2001, states that "large numbers of people must participate in a prevention strategy for direct benefit to relatively few."

In the context of sugar-sweetened beverage taxation, it means that there is some truth in the grumblings of people who argue, "I do not have a weight problem, and the government should not infringe upon my rights."

Yes, but the reason bans can work is because with the ban, some people stop and consider whether they actually need a two-liter bottle of juice–and whether they are willing to pay more to have it now. For people on a budget–these negative incentives raise awareness and promote small behavior changes as seen in Philadelphia. Small changes can morph into lifestyle patterns that have a large effect on the environment and culture around obesity.

However, the most important reason that population-wide prevention measures work for obesity is because they can prevent the development of obesity in the first place. One of the most compelling arguments posed by medicine and public health agencies is that taxation can interrupt the alarming rise in childhood obesity.

I had a firsthand look at the origins of socioeconomic disparities in childhood obesity when we enrolled our child in a home-based daycare because it was much less costly than its commercial counterpart. Our daycare provider received subsidies from the state because she was serving a large population of low-income children. She used those subsidies to purchase food and beverages for the children.

During snack time, she served chips and juice to the children. Alarm bells went off for our family. The absence of policies restricting the use of state funds to feed children was a missed opportunity to avert bad lifestyle habits. Had there been a tax in place on sugared beverages, I wonder whether her purchasing patterns, and the children's consumption patterns, would have changed.

We were able to move our son to a private university–run daycare that followed recommendations from the American Academy of Pediatrics to restrict sugared beverages from children, because we could afford to pay four times more for childcare.

Lower income and even middle-income families with children at the highest risk for obesity should not have to expose their children to obesigenic environments that will compromise their future health. When overweight children grow into obese adults, cycles of obesity and poverty continue because obese adults are subject to discriminatory hiring practices, lower salaries and restricted access to higher-status occupations, which ultimately limits their economic potential.

To be certain, there are multiple factors contributing to obesity. Focusing solely on food ignores the role that sedentary behaviors, short and poor-quality sleep and stressful lifestyles have on obesity. Further, as we learned in the Flint water crisis, water is not always a safe beverage.

Despite significant pushback from individuals and even entire cities like the city of Chicago where I live that repealed a sugar-beverage tax shortly after its rollout, I remain convinced that these population-wide approaches are our best weapon against the epidemic of obesity.

However, a balanced portfolio of policies that attack "sinful" behaviors and promote "virtuous" behaviors will be most effective. Subsidizing healthy choices and providing access to those choices shifts the focus from what you cannot do to what you should–and provides specific guidance.

Policies and regulations targeting the environment are the least personally stigmatizing because they do not blame individuals for poor choices. Rather, they focus on creating environments where the healthy choice becomes the easy choice.

And that is no small matter.

The views expressed are those of the author(s) and are not necessarily those of Scientific American.

About the Author

Mercedes Carnethon, PhD, FAHA, is the Mary Harris Thompson Professor of Preventive Medicine and chief of the Division of Epidemiology at the Feinberg School of Medicine at Northwestern University and a Public Voices Fellow through The OpEd Project.

The Opioid Epidemic Is Surging among Black People because of Unequal Access to Treatment

By Melba Newsome and Gioncarlo Valentine

In one way or another, Thomas Gooch has spent more than 30 years struggling with illegal drugs. The 52-year-old Nashville, Tenn., native grew up in extreme poverty. He was first incarcerated in 1988 and spent the next 15 years in and out of jail for using and selling narcotics. "Until 2003," Gooch says. "That was the first time I went to treatment and the last time I used." Since then, for most of 19 years, Gooch has been trying to get others into recovery or just keep them alive. He handed out clean needles and injection-drug equipment–which reduce injuries, infections and overdose deaths–in Nashville's hardest-hit communities. In 2014 he founded My Father's House, a transitional recovery facility for fathers struggling with substance use disorder.

But despite Gooch's long experience, the opioid epidemic recently has brought a level of devastation to the Black community that has shocked him. "I had never seen death the way I've seen death when it comes to opioid addiction," he says. "There's been so many funerals, it doesn't even make sense. I personally know at least 50 to 60 individuals who died from overdoses in the last 10 years." That staggering body count includes Gooch's recently estranged wife in 2020 and a former partner in 2019.

A million people in the U.S. have died of opioid overdoses since the 1990s. But the face–and race–of the opioid epidemic has changed in the past decade. Originally white and middle class, victims are now Black and brown people struggling with long-term addictions and too few resources. During 10 brutal years, opioid and stimulant deaths have increased 575 percent among Black Americans. In 2019 the overall drug overdose death rate among Black people exceeded that of whites for the first time: 36.8 versus

31.6 per 100,000. And with the addition of fentanyl, the synthetic opioid that's 50 to 100 times more powerful than morphine, Black men older than 55 who survived for decades with a heroin addiction are dying at rates four times greater than people of other races in that age group.

The reasons for this dramatic change come down to racial inequities. Research shows that Black people have a harder time getting into treatment programs than white people do, and Black people are less likely to be prescribed the gold standard medications for substance use therapy. "If you are a Black person and have an opioid use disorder, you are likely to receive treatment five years later than if you're a white person," says Nora D. Volkow, director of the National Institute on Drug Abuse at the National Institutes of Health. "Treatments are extraordinarily useful in terms of preventing overdose death so you can actually recover. Five years can make the difference between being alive or not." Black people with substance use problems are afraid of being caught up in a punitive criminal justice system and are less likely to have insurance good enough to allow them to seek help on their own. And the COVID pandemic disrupted many recovery and harm-reduction services, particularly for people of color.

Gooch blames straight-out racial discrimination in the health-care system, too. "When we call different places to try to get people into treatment, the question they ask is 'What drug do they use?'" he recounts with exasperation. "If you say 'crack,' all of a sudden they ain't got no bed available. If you say opioids and heroin, they will find a bed because that's the demographic they want. A couple of times I told patients that the only way they're going to get help is to get drunk and turn themselves into Vanderbilt Hospital because Vanderbilt will hold them for five days, and that'll get them into treatment."

Gooch is one of the people trying to improve access to therapies for addiction and change the overall dysfunctional dynamic. Other groups are bringing more effective addiction treatments within prison walls, reducing the chances of recidivism on release. A proposed federal law would make therapy with the commonly used addiction medication methadone less onerous for an impoverished population, as well as less stigmatizing. And Volkow is using her platform at the NIH to highlight the overwhelming research-based evidence for better ways to understand and treat addiction.

Access to Treatment

The nation's historic reluctance to treat addiction as a health-care issue rather than a criminal justice one has resulted in a health-care system where too few people of any race—just 10 percent—receive treatment for substance use disorder. Several factors, such as stigma and an inability to afford or access care, make the numbers considerably more dismal among people of color. Even after a nonfatal overdose, Black patients are half as likely to be referred to or access treatment as non-Hispanic white patients, according to federal government data.

A growing recognition that criminalization and incarceration do little to curb illegal drug use or improve public health or safety has led to harm-reduction policies such as Good Samaritan laws—statutes that provide limited immunity for low-level drug violations and increase availability of naloxone, a drug that can reverse overdose. But racial disparities have emerged in the application and effectiveness of both measures. A study from RTI International found that Black and Latino intravenous drug users have inequitable access to the medication.

Loftin Wilson, program manager for the NC Harm Reduction Coalition in Durham, N.C., who has worked in the field for more than a decade, says the problems with inequality lead to distrust in the system, which creates a vicious cycle in which people who need help won't go to institutions that can provide help. People entering treatment worry, with good reason, that dealing with the social service system can cause them to lose their employment, housing or even custody of their children. "That's another example of the negative experiences people who use drugs have. They definitely don't land equally on everybody, and people don't experience them all the same way. It is a vastly different experience to be a Black drug user seeking health care than for a white person," Wilson says.

University of Cincinnati psychologist Kathleen Burlew notes, as Volkow does, that when Black patients enter treatment, they are more likely to do so later than white people and are less likely to complete it. In addition to mistrust, she says, the less favorable outcomes result from factors such as clinician bias and lack of racial and ethnic diversity among treatment providers.

Federal resources, such as grants to support local opioid use disorder clinics and programs, also tend to favor white populations. According to 2021 data from the Substance Abuse and Mental Health Services Administration, 77 percent of the clients treated with grant funding were white, 12.9 percent were Black and 2.8 percent were Native American. The disparity is even more pronounced in some states. For example, in 2019 North Carolina announced that white people made up 88 percent of those served by its $54-million federal grant, compared with 7.5 percent for Black people. Native Americans accounted for less than 1 percent of those served.

Medication Inequality

Research has shown that there is a bias among health-care providers against using medication-assisted treatment (MAT), which combines FDA-approved drugs with counseling and behavioral therapies. Substance use specialists consider it the best approach to the opioid use problem. Yet a study published in *JAMA Network* found that about 40 percent of the 368 U.S. residential drug programs surveyed did not offer MAT, and 21 percent actively discouraged people from using it. Many addiction treatment programs are faith-based and see addiction as a moral problem, which leads to the conclusion that relying on medication for abstinence or sobriety simply trades one form of addiction for another. Many general practitioners who lack training in addiction medicine have this misconception.

The three medications approved by the FDA are buprenorphine, methadone and naltrexone. Buprenorphine and methadone are synthetic opioids that block brain opioid receptors and reduce both cravings and withdrawal. Naltrexone is a postdetox monthly injectable that blocks the effects of opioids. Very few insurance providers in the U.S. cover all three medications, and according to the Centers for Disease Control and Prevention, the full range of medications is far less available to Black people.

Research suggests that economics and race influence who receives which medications. Buprenorphine, for instance, is more widely available in counties with predominantly white communities, whereas methadone clinics are usually located in poor communities of color.

To use methadone, patients must make daily visits to a clinic to receive and take the medication under the supervision of a practitioner. This requirement makes it difficult to do things that build a normal life, such as attending school and obtaining and maintaining a job. There is also the stigma of standing in a public line known to everyone passing by as a queue for addiction treatment. "The treatment model was developed [during the Nixon administration] based on racism and a stigmatized view of people with addiction without any thought of privacy or dignity or treating addiction like a health problem," says Andrew Kolodny, medical director of the Opioid Policy Research Collaborative at Brandeis University. The stigma is made worse by methadone's classification as a Schedule II controlled substance, which is defined as a substance with a high potential for abuse, potentially leading to severe psychological or physical dependence. This categorization pushed the medication into a quasicriminalized status and the clinics into minority communities.

Buprenorphine, however, is a completely different story. When opioid use problems increased in white communities, Congress acted to create less stigmatizing treatment options. The Drug Addiction Treatment Act of 2000 ("DATA 2000") lifted an 86-year ban that prevented treating opioid addiction with narcotic medications such as buprenorphine, which today is sold under the brand names Subutex and Suboxone. The majority of doctors who got special federal licenses to prescribe it accept only commercial health insurance and cash, so the drug is usually offered to a more affluent population, which in the U.S. means white people. About 95 percent of buprenorphine patients are white, and 34 percent have private insurance, according to a national study of data through 2015.

John Woodyear is an addiction treatment specialist in Troy, a small rural town in south central North Carolina where the epidemic is exacting an increasingly heavy toll on the Black and Native American populations. Overall overdose death rates increased 40 percent from 2019 to 2020, but death rates among those two groups in particular went up 66 and 93 percent, respectively. Yet Woodyear, who is Black and practices in a town that is 31 percent Black, says his patients are 90 percent white. People come to the clinic through word of mouth or referrals from friends. As long as Woodyear's patients are mostly white, new patients will be mostly white as well, he says.

One exception to this racial pattern is Edwin Chapman's clinic in the Northeast neighborhood of Washington, D.C., one of the district's predominantly Black and most impoverished communities. Chapman, a physician, often prescribes buprenorphine to his patients with opioid use problems, and the overwhelming majority of them are Black. He says that to prescribe the drug, physicians like him must get past certain roadblocks. "The insurance companies in many states put more restrictions on patients in an urban setting, such as requiring prior authorization for addiction treatment," he says. Further, "to increase the dose above 16 or 24 milligrams, you may have to get a prior authorization. The dosing standards were based on the white population and people who were addicted to pills. Our surviving Black population often needs a higher dose of buprenorphine."

Chapman says few physicians in private practice are willing to treat these patients. "They don't really feel comfortable having these patients in their office, or they aren't really prepared to deal with the economic and mental health issues that come with this population," he explains; those disorders include bipolar disorder and schizophrenia, among others.

People have their own biases that keep them away from medication such as buprenorphine, Wilson says. Many view it as simply trading one drug for another. "They think, 'If I'm going to take this step, why not just go to detox and not take any medications at all?'" he says. "There's a big cultural misunderstanding about the fact that [these] medications are the only evidence-based treatment for opioid use disorder. Short-term detox isn't the most appropriate intervention for most people."

Gooch agrees that the bias is real. He facilitates recovery groups at a program operated by a group from Meharry Medical College, a historically Black institution. Yet "I haven't seen one Black person yet," Gooch says. "Some think it's a setup. There's so much distrust, they have a hard time thinking it's legal. It's just the culture of Black people. Many are religious and think [taking the drug] is wrong."

"Those [misconceptions] are holdovers from our having been miseducated from the outset," Chapman says. "Whites have done a tremendous job educating their community that this is a medical problem, a disease. In the African American community, drug addiction has always been and continues to be seen as a moral problem, and incarceration was the treatment."

Hope for Change

In the November 2021 issue of *Neuropsychopharmacology*, Volkow argued that it is long past time for a new approach to drug addiction that would address these misconceptions within the most affected populations and biases among providers. "We have known for decades that addiction is a medical condition–a treatable brain disorder–not a character flaw or a form of social deviance," she wrote.

Volkow argues that treatment reform should start with prison and the criminal justice system. Even though there is no difference along racial lines in who uses illegal drugs, Black people nonetheless were arrested for drug offenses at five times the rate of white people in 2016. The racial disproportionality in incarcerated drug offenders does not reflect higher rates of drug law violations, only higher rates of arrest among racial and ethnic minorities. Currently the number of arrests for heroin (which more Black people use) exceeds the arrests for diverted prescription opioids (which more white people use), even though the latter is more prevalent.

These unequal arrests and incarcerations add to the racial inequalities in drug treatment and survival rates. An estimated two thirds of people in U.S. correctional settings have a diagnosable substance use disorder, and approximately 95 percent will relapse after their release. In the two weeks postrelease, the risk of overdose increases more than 100-fold, and the chances of death increase 12-fold.

Paradoxically, that makes prisons and jails–institutions with the most obvious and overt racial disparities–the places with the greatest potential to bring about effective change. Volkow points to a recent NIH study as proof that starting substance disorder treatment during incarceration lowers the risk of probation violations and reincarcerations and improves the chances of recovery. But only one in 13 prisoners with substance use problems receives treatment, according to a Pew data analysis.

Some local programs have started to tackle some of these issues. In Pittsburgh, the Allegheny Health Network's RIvER (Rethinking Incarceration and Empowering Recovery) Clinic opened in May 2021. Its goal is to reduce recidivism among people with addictions by providing care for the formerly incarcerated immediately on their release from jail, regardless of their ability to pay. Since opening, the clinic's caregivers have engaged with hundreds of people.

New York City recently became the first municipality in the country to sanction overdose prevention centers where people with substance use disorder can use drugs under medical supervision. Two sites, one in East Harlem and the other in Washington Heights, opened in December 2021. They have had more than 10,000 visits and prevented nearly 200 overdoses by administering the medication naloxone.

There are other signs of change, too. California signed a law that requires every treatment provider in the state to provide a "client bill of rights" to notify patients of all aspects of recommended treatment, including no treatment at all, treatment risks and expected results. And federal authorities loosened methadone regulations during the pandemic. Instead of daily in-person visits, more patients were allowed to use telehealth consultations and take doses home. Senators Ed Markey of Massachusetts and Rand Paul of Kentucky have introduced a bill that would make that change permanent. Among other programs and initiatives across the country, these are an indication that drug treatment policy may be headed in a more equitable, evidence-based direction.

About the Authors

Melba Newsome is an award-winning science, health and environmental reporter. She lives in Charlotte, N.C.

Gioncarlo Valentine is an award-winning photographer and writer from Baltimore. Backed by his seven years of social work experience, Valentine examines issues faced by marginalized populations, most often focusing his lens on the experiences of Black and LGBTQIA+ communities.

Doctors Need to Learn to Talk about Suicide

By Rodolfo Bonnin and Leonard M. Gralnik

The numbers are stark when it comes to suicide: It is a leading cause of death in the United States, and was the second leading cause of death in the U.S. for people ages 10 to 14 and 25 to 34 in 2020. That year, millions of American adults thought of, planned or attempted suicide, and nearly 46,000 died by suicide according to the Centers for Disease Control and Prevention.

Most people who take their own life receive services in primary care and other medical settings in the year prior to death. This raises many critical questions: Did the doctor note any overt or subtle signs of suicidal ideation? Did the doctor discuss suicide with the patient? And if not, why not? Was the doctor uncomfortable broaching the subject? Did they feel unprepared to talk about suicide? Was the patient hesitant to bring it up? If so, was there something about the doctor-patient interaction that led to the patient's hesitancy?

We are a board-certified academic psychiatrist (Gralnik) and a psychologist experienced in training clinicians (Bonnin) who have witnessed patients, practicing physicians, residents and students struggle with this topic. In our experience, as well as that of others, doctors in many specialties have difficulty asking important questions about suicide because of the long history of stigma, stereotypes and misunderstandings about this topic. This must change.

To that end, we have implemented an innovative training program at Florida International University's Herbert Wertheim College of Medicine that is embedded throughout all four years of the curriculum. The significance of this training is that it is a required component of several medical school courses–in contrast to wellness programs, which are usually voluntary and designed to offer emotional support for students. While wellness programs may help medical students to manage their own feelings of depression, helplessness and hopelessness, they don't give them the skills needed to talk to their future patients about suicide. In our training program, sessions beginning in the first year of medical school instruct students about the prevalence of suicide, actively train them in how to interview suicidal patients and help them develop empathy as a fundamentally important clinical skill. Students also participate in interactive sessions where they role-play as a patient and as a clinician assessing a suicidal patient and creating a safety plan.

Based on our experience, doctors sometimes are more awkward than empathetic, beginning this conversation with a preamble or even an apology: for example, "This may seem like a strange question," "I have to ask you a question that we ask all patients" or "I'm sorry if this question seems too personal." These types of statements, while meant to put the patient at ease, may actually increase their anxiety, reinforcing the idea that suicide is a taboo subject. How can we expect our patients to be forthcoming in disclosing their suicidal thoughts if we, as doctors, remain apprehensive about the subject?

Significant training about suicide usually does not begin until the third year of medical school, during psychiatric rotations in clinical settings, which gives the message that this subject is of limited importance to doctors in nonpsychiatric fields. Limiting training about suicide to psychiatric rotations also perpetuates the misconception that suicide occurs only in the context of a diagnosed mental illness We think that all required clinical rotations, including surgery, pediatrics, internal medicine, neurology, family medicine, and obstetrics and gynecology should incorporate enhanced training about suicide.

By including training about suicide as a fully integrated part of the curriculum, we can reduce stigma, and the topic of suicide becomes viewed as an essential part of medical training. The training also includes information about suicide as it affects medical students, residents and practicing physicians, who have high rates of anxiety, burnout and depression. It is ironic that medical students often neglect their own mental health struggles even while receiving training about psychiatric disorders.

Our long-term objective is to prepare all doctors and other medical professionals to discuss suicide openly with their patients, paving the way to better patient care and safety. As we have implemented this curriculum, we have witnessed a significant increase in the comfort level, confidence and competency of students when interviewing real patients with suicidal thoughts.

Because many suicidal people initially visit a doctor who is not a psychiatrist, it is crucial that doctors in other specialties be prepared to detect suicidal ideation, evaluate the person and take appropriate actions. Patients may feel intimidated talking to their doctor about suicide and may be more comfortable when speaking with a physician assistant, nurse or medical assistant. It is crucial that these health care professionals also receive adequate training about suicide assessment and prevention.

To see any tangible change in suicide prevention in the foreseeable future, implementation of enhanced suicide-training programs in all medical schools should begin now. Continuing medical education on this topic also needs to be developed and implemented to train current practicing physicians, and to maintain the clinical skills related to suicide assessment and prevention for future graduates.

A new number for the service formerly called the National Suicide Prevention Lifeline was activated recently: 988 replaces the old number, 1-800-273-8255 (TALK), for what is now the 988 Suicide & Crisis Lifeline. The much simpler three-digit number is a long-overdue step in the right direction toward helping those in need. Providing easier access to crisis intervention services and raising awareness about suicide are important, but there remains a real need to improve doctors' skills when dealing with individuals with suicidal ideation.

The goal of the American Foundation for Suicide Prevention is to reduce by 20 percent the annual suicide rate in the U.S. by 2025. Suicide is preventable, but this will require a shift in medical education. We still have a long way to go.

IF YOU NEED HELP If you or someone you know is struggling or having thoughts of suicide, help is available. Call the 988 Suicide & Crisis Lifeline at 988, use the online Lifeline Chat or contact the Crisis Text Line by texting TALK to 741741.

About the Author

Rodolfo Bonnin received his Ph.D. in counseling psychology from the University of Missouri. He completed his internship training at Florida State University. Bonnin is an associate professor in the department of psychiatry and behavioral health, an assistant dean and director of assessment and evaluation at Florida International University's Herbert Wertheim College of Medicine. He is also a course co-director for professional behavior courses at the college.

Leonard M. Gralnik received his Ph.D. and M.D. from the University of Miami School of Medicine. He completed residency and fellowship training in general psychiatry and child and adolescent psychiatry at the University of Miami/Jackson Memorial Hospital. He is board-certified in general psychiatry and in child and adolescent psychiatry. Gralnik is currently an assistant professor of psychiatry and behavioral health, director of the psychiatry clerkship and chief of psychiatry education at Florida International University's (FIU's) Herbert Wertheim College of Medicine. He is also the senior medical director of the FIU Health Psychiatry Faculty Group Practice. He is a co-author, with Douglas Flemons, of a book on suicide assessment, Relational Suicide Assessment: Risks, Resources and Possibilities for Safety *(Norton Professional Books, 2013).*

Why Does Ebola Keep Showing Up in the Democratic Republic of the Congo?

By Dina Fine Maron

When news broke this week [May 2018] that the Democratic Republic of the Congo is facing yet another Ebola outbreak, many public health experts were not surprised. The vast central African country has dealt with more outbreaks of this often-fatal hemorrhagic disease than any other nation. Yet exactly why the DRC is hit so often remains an unanswered question.

The DRC Ministry of Health announced the latest outbreak this week after laboratory testing confirmed two cases had occurred in the northwestern part of the country, near the its border with the similarly named Republic of the Congo. This is DRC's ninth Ebola outbreak since scientists first identified the disease.

Most of the country's outbreaks burn out quickly because they occur in relatively remote areas—but each has had a high fatality rate. The world's first-known Ebola cases occurred in the DRC in 1976 (when the country was called Zaire), killing 280 of the 318 people known to have been infected. Last year eight cases were reported, and half of the infected people died.

The disease spreads among humans through direct contact with the bodily fluids of a person who is sick with or has died from Ebola. It can be transmitted via sexual contact. It can also spread to people who encounter the bodily fluids or viscera of infected primates or bats, such as when someone prepares these animals for food. Most outbreaks have originated in Africa or from lab accidents elsewhere, and have remained small—but people traveling from sites of a 2014 outbreak that roiled west Africa led to isolated cases in locations including the U.K., Italy, Spain and the U.S.

Ebola experts have various suspicions about why the DRC remains so vulnerable. Most theories involve the country's large forested areas, and the possibility that infected fruit bats—widely believed to be the primary reservoir animal for the disease–are common in the affected areas. "If you live or work in a forest where bats roost, you may have the bad luck to be in touch with bat guano from an infected animal. Or perhaps you encountered saliva or guano on a piece of fruit which an infected fruit bat was involved with," says Daniel Bausch, a veteran Ebola responder and director of the U.K. Public Health Rapid Support Team. In certain areas of the DRC–including where Ebola has been reported recently–the disease can now be considered endemic in reservoir animals, he says.

During the massive Ebola crisis that gripped west Africa from 2014 to 2016, researchers were told about a bat-filled roosting tree in Guinea they suspected may have been ground zero for that outbreak. Rounding up some of those bats could have given scientists a chance to test the animals and confirm them as a main reservoir for the disease. But the tree burned down and the bats were reduced to char, destroying the opportunity to search for much evidence–although researchers were able to use trace DNA fragments to pinpoint that they were *Mops condylurus*, an insect-eating species common across central and west Africa.

Whether experts will be able to find infected bats during the latest DRC outbreak remains unknown, partly because there may have been undetected cases of the disease dating back months; any culprit bat colony may have moved on by now. "If the outbreak started last month, then yes, it would be interesting to sample the bats. But if it started in December, then no, the best thing to do may be come to back next December" (when the same type of bats may return to the area), says Pierre Rollin, an Ebola expert at the U.S. Centers for Disease Control and Prevention who has responded to most known Ebola outbreaks.

Peter Piot, director of the London School of Hygiene and Tropical Medicine, who was part of the team that originally discovered the virus in 1976, also believes people's interactions with infected bats may be behind the repeated outbreaks there. "Due to its huge swathes of forest, the DRC is a reservoir for the virus, making the country particularly susceptible to outbreaks of Ebola," he says.

"Occasionally people living in these rural areas will come into contact with infected animals, and the transmission cycle begins." Some experts also suspect deforestation could be a factor, bringing infected animals and people together in the area when they may cut down trees or butcher infected bats for food. DRC is about the size of Greenland–almost a million square miles–and much of it has long been forested, notes Peter Hotez, dean of the National School of Tropical Medicine at Baylor College of Medicine.

The extent to which individual countries can detect, confirm and report the disease may also affect scientists' understanding of why it occurs where it does. Whether or not the DRC is truly seeing the disease much more than some of its neighbors is debatable, Rollin says. "I think there could be surveillance bias–it's difficult to say," he says, noting the neighboring Republic of the Congo had multiple Ebola outbreaks in the early 2000s, although none have been reported since 2003. "The reservoir [animal] is in DRC, Gabon and the Republic of [the] Congo," he says. So what's different? The DRC has more robust Ebola surveillance and lab testing capacity in place, he says, and that may be a factor.

The U.K.'s rapid response team and the CDC are both standing by to help respond to the latest outbreak, and are consulting with the World Health Organization and the DRC's Ministry of Health. But the British and U.S. organizations are not yet part of the formal response on the ground. The formal response team–WHO, Doctors Without Borders and the DRC health ministry–have just arrived in the area, Rollin says, so there are still many unknowns.

In the latest DRC outbreak, "it is concerning that of the 21 reported cases so far, 17 are fatal. That makes me think this is the tip of the iceberg. But how large the iceberg is right now, it's too early to say. It is appropriate to be taking this seriously and mounting a firm response," Bausch says. "The village at the heart of the current outbreak is remote by land but it is on a major river with access to major population centers via the water route. And there is always concern about connections between populations."

About the Author

Dina Fine Maron, formerly an associate editor at Scientific American, *is now a wildlife trade investigative reporter at* National Geographic.

Ebola Outbreak in Uganda Surges, but the Country Has a Plan

By Paul Adepoju

A 24-year-old man who tested positive for Ebola virus disease caused by *Sudan ebolavirus* (SUDV) was the first confirmed case in Uganda's ongoing Ebola outbreak, but health authorities believe he was probably not the initial, or index, case. As of October 9, confirmed cases totaled 48, with 17 deaths, according to the Ministry of Health Uganda. But those numbers will likely continue to rise.

Uganda's health authorities officially declared the outbreak on September 20. An approved vaccine for Ebola exists, but it is not effective against SUDV, the strain responsible for the outbreak. Several vaccines are in various stages of development against this strain, two of which could begin clinical trials in Uganda in the coming weeks, pending regulatory and ethics approvals from the Ugandan government and availability of doses for the trial. One is a single-dose vaccine that was developed by the Sabin Vaccine Institute. The other was developed by the University of Oxford's Jenner Institute.

Although health authorities have attempted to reassure the public despite the lack of approved vaccines, the deaths of at least four health workers–including a doctor and a midwife–are raising concerns about the safety of frontline health workers who are responding to the outbreak.

Patrick Otim, health emergency officer of the Acute Events Management Unit at the World Health Organization's Regional Office for Africa, says the response relies on the continual cooperation of the affected communities and the responders. So far community members have been cooperating, Otim says. "The teams that are [in] the field are receiving cooperation from the community in terms of investigation, listing of contacts and referral of suspected cases," he says.

According to Uganda's Ministry of Health, as of October 9, 1049 people who have been in contact with an infected person had been listed for follow-up, while 14 active cases had been admitted to the hospital for monitoring.

To prevent further spread, the response strategy prioritizes quickly identifying and isolating infected people, managing their care in treatment centers, engaging the community so that individuals can take preventive measures and ensuring that people comply with the public health interventions. "We believe that, by implementing these measures this time, [we should be] able to contain the outbreak without having much further transmission," Otim says.

Scientific American spoke with Kyobe Henry Bbosa, Ebola incident commander at Uganda's Ministry of Health, about the outbreak's spread, as well as the country's preparedness, response and public health strategies.

[An edited transcript of the interview follows.]

Q: What do we know about how and when the outbreak started?

A: The epidemic seems to have started around early September, when people started dying in villages in the Madudu and Kiruma subcounties in central Uganda. The person with the first confirmed case presented to a regional referral hospital with symptoms of the disease after being treated in several places. Since we identified the SUDV at the Uganda Virus Research Institute, additional cases have been confirmed. The cases have come mainly from five subcounties in central Uganda's Mubende district. We are also investigating cases that may have come from another neighboring district.

Q: How does the epicenter of the current outbreak compare with that of previous ones?

A: The district lies on a major highway that leads into Kampala [the capital of Uganda] from the Democratic Republic of the Congo. It has busy trading places and a gold mine on one side, very close to the current epicenter of the outbreak. Uganda has had a number of SUDV outbreaks. The first was in 2000, when we had more than 200 deaths. The second one happened in 2012 in central Uganda, a bit farther away from this outbreak. And now we have the current one. Since the first one, we have gained significant expertise to be able to respond to this disease.

Q: How has the COVID pandemic contributed to preparedness and response?

A: This current outbreak is happening just at the end of the peak of the COVID pandemic, which we think we managed successfully. We are quickly repurposing some of the infrastructure we used for COVID for Ebola. We now have significant capacity built across the country for protection and also to be able to galvanize committed support for a response. So we think that, using what we have done before, we should be able to appropriately respond to the current outbreak.

We have identified contacts, we are continuing to do contact tracing, and we are repurposing and extending the treatment center that had actually previously been used for COVID and enhancing public awareness.

Q: What is the outlook for the outbreak? Is there a risk of cross-border transmission?

A: The 72 hours following the confirmation of the first case showed this is a rapidly evolving picture–very complex–the full extent and scope of which we don't yet know. We think cases may rise in a few days without our full knowledge of the extent of contacts. But we're working so much with the collaboration of other local and international partners to make sure that we care for people, that we ensure the safety of our health workers and, of course, that we bring this to an end as soon as possible so that we can protect our neighbor countries, and they don't have to deal with cross-border transmission.

Q: What do we know about what is driving the outbreak and its geographical reach?

A: Our investigations have not yet been able to identify the index case. We almost certainly know the virus was transmitted from a wild animal into the human population. Some hypotheses have been proposed relating to the country's mango season. We are at the end of the mango season when people–mostly children–start to eat whatever they find [including fruit contaminated by an infected animal]. These are hypotheses that we are trying to work through to understand the origin of the outbreak and certainly find the index case. But we are currently primarily focused on contact tracing, caring for patients, protecting health care workers and providing information to people to prevent further spread.

This particular outbreak is most likely a spillover from wildlife. We have no evidence of this strain of Ebola virus in the recent past to suspect it came from a different outbreak. The last Ebola [Sudan ebolavirus] outbreak that happened in Sudan was more than 10 years ago, and we think it is much less likely to be a spillover from that. We think this is a fresh spillover from the wild into the human population, where it is currently circulating.

As for the geographical distribution, the main epicenter of the outbreak is Mubende district, which is near the center of Uganda. But within that, we have five subcounties [where cases have mainly occurred]. We are looking at a span of 70 kilometers from one end to the other. For the disease clusters within the subcounties, we are looking at a distance of up to 30 km. The breadth of response is the whole country. We are hoping to extend the response across the 11 districts surrounding the one at the epicenter.

Q: Why did it take so long for the health authorities to flag the outbreak?

A: There is a little bit of time lag from what we think is a probable case to a real case. We can't determine the index case until we confirm it. Ebola resembles most of the other tropical diseases such as malaria and typhoid. Initially, its presentation in the local setting appeared to be like other illnesses, and that contributed to a little bit of a delay. But as soon as the first confirmed case came to a major facility, we were able to diagnose Ebola.

This was, in a way, expected, largely because the individuals were mainly moving from one private health facility to the other seeking care. It was only when they reported to public health facilities that we were able to make a diagnosis.

Q: With no approved vaccine for this strain, what is the plan to protect frontline health workers?

A: Those who are working in highly infectious settings have different sets of PPE [personal protective equipment] from those who are working in other areas of the hospital facilities. We have a sufficient amount of PPE. The WHO deployed an Ebola kit, which we are now using in the management of Ebola patients. But in addition, we still have leftover kits from COVID that we are still using.

About the Author

Paul Adepoju is a science journalist based in Nigeria.

"Their Lives Are Worth More Than Ours": Experts in Africa Slam Global Response to Monkeypox

By Paul Adepoju

World Health Organization (WHO) director general Tedros Adhanom Ghebreyesus has now officially declared monkeypox a public health emergency of international concern (PHEIC). The decision comes after the global health body's International Health Regulations Emergency Committee on the disease failed to reach a consensus on the declaration at the end of its second meeting in less than a month. Between the meetings, the number of confirmed cases worldwide rose from 3,040 across 47 countries to more than 16,000 in 75 countries and territories, and the number of deaths rose from one to five, according to the WHO.

Before a PHEIC was declared, Matshidiso Moeti, WHO regional director for Africa, told *Scientific American* that earlier action would have drawn additional attention to the disease and spurred countries to assess the risks and be better prepared. She added that it would also have made more funding and resources available to African countries–where monkeypox has been endemic for decades–to respond to the disease.

An earlier declaration had the potential to "trigger additional attention from all countries, and possibly then trigger the availability and the allocation of additional resources at the global level that might be available to African countries," Moeti said. "It places an obligation on some of the entities that control some of the tools available to provide support."

Tedros thinks it isn't too late, however. In his PHEIC declaration, he said that "with the tools we have right now, we can stop transmission and bring this outbreak under control."

In the Democratic Republic of the Congo (DRC), additional resources could have helped expand response efforts to many provinces that had suspected cases but were not being supported by current partners, according to Justin Masumu, dean of the faculty of veterinary medicine at DRC's National Pedagogical University.

Moeti noted to *Scientific American* that the WHO is working with African countries and has been providing all available support. But Christian Happi, director of African Center of Excellence for Genomics of Infectious Diseases, disagrees with some aspects of the WHO's handling of the monkeypox outbreak, describing them as shameful. According to him, there was no talk of using the world's stockpile of smallpox vaccine for monkeypox when cases were only being reported in African countries.

"But today, [now] that they have [monkeypox] in the Global North, they're now mobilizing stuff, and it's a shame [for] the WHO to do that," he says.

According to a spokesperson for the WHO, the organization "continues to work closely with the ministries of health and the laboratory networks in the African region, and supports the countries that have been reporting cases of monkeypox in the last few years such as Nigeria, Democratic Republic of the Congo, Central African Republic and Cameroon."

Stretched, Finite Resources

In Nigeria, monkeypox reemerged in 2017 after nearly 40 years of no confirmed cases. While the number of confirmed cases in the country dropped from a previous peak of 88 in 2017 to just eight in 2020, as of July 17, 2022, the case count has reached 117, according to the Nigeria Center for Disease Control (NCDC).

NCDC's director general Ifedayo Adetifa says the Nigerian government has initiated an emergency response to the current monkeypox outbreak and has had surveillance in place since 2017. But he admits that limited resources pose a challenge to the country's ability to simultaneously respond to multiple disease outbreaks. "We have limited, finite resources that are all being competed for by varying priorities," Adetifa says. "We continue to deal with everything–Lassa fever, cholera, measles, yellow fever, monkeypox [and] COVID–as the case requires, regardless of what the headlines are focused on," he says.

Testing Gaps

Several African countries continue to provide daily updates on the state of the COVID pandemic. But such updates are not available for monkeypox, and a major reason for this is the gap between the number of suspected and confirmed cases. From January 1 to July 8, there were a total of 2,087 suspected monkeypox cases on the continent, of which only 203 were confirmed. This wide gap has been attributed to the paucity of testing kits and ingredients such as reagents.

"While all African countries have the polymerase chain reaction machines needed to test for monkeypox, thanks to reinforced laboratory capacity in the wake of COVID-19, many lack reagents and, in some cases, training in specimen collection, handling and testing," Moeti told Scientific American. She said the WHO is working to secure 60,000 tests for Africa, of which about 2,000 tests and reagents will be shipped to high-risk countries–such as the DRC–that account for about 80 percent of suspected cases on the continent.

Masumu notes that because of inadequate testing, the true magnitude of the monkeypox outbreak in the DRC is not yet known. "What is true is that what we know is not the reality," he says. "We don't analyze all the suspected samples. We should have many more cases in the field that are not recorded."

Vaccine Inequity

Critics have highlighted inequity in the distribution of COVID vaccines as one of the reasons for their low uptake in Africa. A similar trend is already occurring with the distribution of smallpox vaccines, which also protect against monkeypox, according to the Africa Centers for Disease Control and Prevention (Africa CDC).

Had a PHEIC been declared sooner, Moeti noted, African countries could have had access to additional tools, including unapproved vaccines for the disease. But Ahmed Ogwell Ouma, acting director of the Africa CDC, revealed in a press briefing on July 21 that there are no smallpox vaccine doses on the continent.

In sharp contrast, the U.S. government has already distributed more than 191,000 doses of vaccines in response to monkeypox. On July 15 it added 131,000 doses of Bavarian Nordic's JYNNEOS monkeypox vaccine to its stockpile, and 786,000 more doses are expected by the end of the month. The country also has about 100 million doses of ACAM2000, a Food and Drug Administration–licensed vaccine for smallpox that also works against monkeypox but has side effects and should not be used in immunocompromised people. (The U.S. response to monkeypox has not been perfect, however.)

A similar vaccination rollout is also underway in the U.K., which has recently acquired an additional 100,000 vaccine doses to continue its selective vaccine strategy–an approach that aims to interrupt "transmission in the subset of individuals at increased risk," according to the U.K. Health Security Agency. This includes gay, bisexual or other men who have sex with men.

Happi argues that while a prompt emergency declaration backed with a holistic approach to tackle the disease everywhere would have been a sound public health strategy, the current inequity will further put global health at risk.

"Our lives are not the same; their lives are worth more than ours," Happi says, referring to people in African nations versus those in wealthy Western countries. "But unfortunately for them, because you think you're [only] neglecting some other people, you will keep having the disease in your backyard, you will keep struggling with it. Any outbreak anywhere should concern the whole world, [which is] not how they are dealing with it now."

The Bigger Picture

Happi believes that the current impasse should drive Africa to rally behind the Africa CDC to meet the continent's public health emergency response needs. "The reason why people are reckoning with Africa CDC is because [the agency is] very pragmatic. [It's] very impactful," he says.

The Executive Council of the African Union agrees. At a recent meeting, it adopted an amended statute of the Africa CDC that empowers the health agency to declare public health emergencies of continental security concern even when the WHO doesn't declare a PHEIC. The WHO initially pushed back against this amendment because of its concern that such a declaration could potentially result in travel restrictions similar to the travel bans that were announced when South Africa's genomic surveillance network first reported the Omicron variant of SARS-CoV-2, the virus responsible for COVID-19.

Similarly, Karim Tounkara, regional representative for Africa at the World Organization for Animal Health, says that in order to have a better response to monkeypox and other zoonotic diseases, African countries need to prioritize prevention. And this can be done by countries better appropriating the "One Health" approach that treats human, animal and environmental health as interconnected and paying more attention to wildlife monitoring to prevent future outbreaks.

"We encourage all countries to do everything possible to strengthen the capacity for early detection and early response," Tounkara says. In addition to improving testing among the population, he says, attention should be given to strengthening the capacity of veterinary diagnostic laboratories because "it will always be better to tackle the disease from the animal sources."

About the Author

Paul Adepoju is a science journalist based in Nigeria.

We Can't Let Monkeypox Turn into a Repeat of COVID

By Muhammad Jawad Noon

Monkeypox is spreading: there have been more than 3,000 confirmed cases of this virus in over 40 countries, and the actual number is likely much higher. Although the monkeypox virus is not normally as contagious or transmissible as coronavirus, this peculiar spread of cases worldwide is worrisome, because there are still so many unknowns.

I had a déjà vu while listening to the WHO's monkeypox briefing on the occasion of the 75th World Health Assembly in May 2022. Amid the uncertainty and the limited understanding of the current outbreak, the WHO cautioned governments to collaborate and act responsibly to stop the virus's transmission. It sounded like an excerpt from 2020 when public health organizations made the same warnings about COVID. I wondered if politicians would respond similarly–disjointedly–ignoring public health messaging. I worried monkeypox would turn into a sequel to COVID.

As a medical doctor who studies policy and economics, I found it gut-wrenching to witness so many governments' disgraceful, and at times fraudulent, responses to COVID. In 2.5 years of this pandemic (no, the pandemic is still not over), with mismanagement of prevention measures and a vaccine effort plagued with misinformation, millions of people have died, many millions more have been sickened and a sizable portion are living with long COVID, and vaccination rates in some countries are dismal.

The global monkeypox outbreak is a test for world leaders. We are still in early days, and policy makers have a small window of opportunity to act quickly and put the right measures in place to stop monkeypox from turning into another disaster. They should strengthen virus surveillance and work on deploying decentralized, privacy-preserving and encrypted contact tracing to avoid data breaches and to ensure trust within their communities. There are many unknowns about this outbreak, and political leaders should avoid making sweeping statements; instead, they should raise public awareness based on information scrutinized by science experts. They should also be prepared to combat the tidal wave of a possible "misinfodemic."

Countries must set up proper testing and molecular diagnostic facilities to detect cases early. In addition, governments should accelerate the monkeypox research agenda and share anonymized data with the WHO using its standardized protocol, so that data can be compared across countries and regions. And importantly, government officials must refrain from stigmatizing people who have monkeypox. COVID has given nations worldwide a literal checklist of what not to do. The question is, how will we proceed this time?

I still remember the early days of COVID confusion. I was in the Frankfurt airport in January 2020, in a line with people who had flown in from China. They were all wearing masks. The World Health Organization's Novel Coronavirus (2019-nCoV) situation report had been published, which mentioned the spread of coronavirus to Japan, the Republic of Korea and Thailand. By that time the Centers for Disease Control and Prevention in the U.S. had also reported the first travel-related case of COVID in that nation.

The WHO struggled in the beginning to be consistent in its messaging–as what we were learning changed in real time and there was a lack of clear evidence on the dynamics of COVID transmission. Politicians, for example, in the U.S. and Japan, did not let it go unnoticed.

They accused the WHO of becoming China's coronavirus accomplice, instead of focusing on the shortcomings of their own response to the pandemic. The WHO had declared COVID a public health emergency of international concern by the end of January. This was the precursor to the official declaration of a pandemic a few weeks later. I would like to pose this question to world leaders: How do they rate their response to COVID after January 30?

In the U.K. and the U.S., for instance, government officials publicly tap-danced around scientists' recommendations for physical distancing and even boasted about doing the opposite. The pandemic became politicized. Political and economic gains overrode public health interests.

I am still unable to fully grasp the rationale behind leaders in office spreading misinformation and promoting unproven coronavirus remedies such as hydroxychloroquine or ivermectin, knowing that people's lives were at stake. The unfortunate cocktail of lies, fake news, politics, blame and incompetent governance during a highly lethal pandemic has put the public on the losing end.

In the U.S. alone, more than 200,000 children lost a parent or caregiver to COVID-19. Research shows that orphans are at greater risk of poverty, substance abuse, suicide and mental health issues. History is filled with examples of politicians able to get away with face-saving tactics, but how long are we going to tolerate this deceit?

Furthermore, the flawed approach to vaccine distribution led to global vaccine inequity and deepened the health crisis. When India and South Africa proposed a temporary intellectual property ban on the COVID vaccine at the World Trade Organization to promote mass production of shots, they were opposed by several high-income countries, citing it as a barrier to innovation. Human Rights Watch called this move "inaccurate, misleading, and misguided." The People's Vaccine Alliance has expressed their concerns over the emergence of vaccine-resistant variants as a result of persistently low vaccine coverage in numerous nations.

At present, the WHO does not recommend mass immunization for monkeypox. Nevertheless, countries are stockpiling; the U.S. has ordered jabs worth $119 million from Denmark's Bavarian Nordic, which is the only company that manufactures a vaccine approved for monkeypox in the U.S. I wholeheartedly support the idea of epidemic preparedness, but my question is, if the monkeypox outbreak gets out of hand, will these countries support global equitable access to the monkeypox vaccine?

Monkeypox is so far less deadly than COVID. Its spread may soon fizzle out. But if it doesn't, government officials all over the world have a responsibility to learn from the mistakes of the COVID pandemic and not repeat them. The transcript of the last 2.5 years is right in front of them. Will they act in defense of public health, or will they, again, indulge in their political acrobatics and be indifferent to human suffering? And will we, as a global population, let our governments treat us this way?

This is an opinion and analysis article, and the views expressed by the author or authors are not necessarily those of Scientific American.

About the Author

Muhammad Jawad Noon is a medical doctor, currently working as a researcher in economic sciences at the University of Göttingen, Germany. He has contributed to Nature, Fortune *and* Al Jazeera, *among other publications. He was the recipient of the German Medical Award 2020 (Academic).*

Section 5: What Lies Ahead

5.1 Tick- and Mosquito-Borne Diseases Are Increasing Dramatically
By Kacey C. Ernst

5.2 Want to Prevent Another Coronavirus Epidemic?
By William A. Haseltine

5.3 The Next Zika
By Marta Zaraska

5.4 COVID Is Here to Stay
By Christine Crudo Blackburn

Tick- and Mosquito-Borne Diseases Are Increasing Dramatically

By Kacey C. Ernst

People celebrate the arrival of summer every year, but it comes with a downside: an annual population explosion of disease-carrying ticks and mosquitoes. Recent findings from the Centers for Disease Control and Prevention reveal a staggering *threefold* increase in reported cases of what we broadly term "vector-borne diseases"—or illnesses transmitted to humans by mosquitoes, lice, ticks and the like—between 2004 and 2016 in the United States. Making matters worse, nine new pathogens emerged for the first time in the U.S. during this same period.

What has spurred such a dramatic uptick (no pun intended)? While multiple factors are involved, the influence of climate change cannot be overlooked.

Climate Change and Disease

Since vectors are cold-blooded, changes in temperature alter both the biology and population dynamics of mosquitos and ticks, which in turn impacts their development rates, feeding patterns and reproductive cycles. When temperatures rise, the time between generations of mosquitoes shortens. What's more, earlier and extended periods of warm weather may prolong the time during which vector populations are able to thrive. (On the flip side, extremely hot temperatures coupled with drier conditions in some areas can have a negative impact on vector populations.)

Disease pathogens are also influenced by weather patterns. For example, the virus that causes dengue fever goes through the developmental stages in the mosquito more rapidly when temperatures are warmer. That means the time it takes from when a mosquito bites an infected person and can pass on the virus is much quicker.

Spring is arriving earlier each year, meaning mosquito and tick populations will grow active earlier along with it. As warm seasons extend, the opportunity for introducing pathogens increases. These conditions, coupled with other human-induced changes, influence risk. For example, cutting away forested areas for suburban development has been identified as a significant contributor to the expansion of Lyme disease in New England.

The precise contribution of climate change to current and future increases in vector-borne diseases within the U.S. is not well-established. Changes in land-use, diagnostics, travel, and importation of goods, combined with flawed data sets, make it difficult to isolate its impact. And some argue that social factors such as indoor lifestyles and good infrastructure (including air conditioning and window screens) will buffer people from the influence climate change might have on vector-borne diseases. What is clear, however, is that these climate-sensitive diseases have a high potential to be influenced by changing weather patterns.

Better Surveillance Needed

We urgently need resources to enhance vector and disease surveillance and to improve our capacity to respond, especially given the uncertainty around how a changing climate may influence the spread of vectors and vector-borne diseases. For diseases transmitted between animal hosts and vectors, like West Nile virus and Lyme disease, monitoring vector populations and non-human hosts may provide an early warning signal to trigger public health responses.

On the other hand, for diseases passed almost exclusively between humans and vectors, such as dengue, virus levels in mosquito populations often coincide with transmission already occurring in humans. Therefore, monitoring mosquito abundance and enhancing our ability to detect human cases is critical.

Community Engagement is Key

Prevention goes hand in glove with detection. While often a secondary public health concern, vector-borne disease prevention efforts made headlines with the spread of the Zika virus in 2015, when it was reported that the virus could have devastating consequences for pregnant women and their babies. However, for many mosquito-borne illnesses threatening the U.S. there is not an effective vaccine or treatment, so the need for better vector-control methods is urgent.

How can communities work together to solve this problem? Part of the answer must include better public education to help people recognize the symptoms of vector-borne diseases. Increased community engagement is also necessary in order to help better understand the specific needs and abilities of that community in regard to public health and vector-control programs.

Some areas are experimenting with new technologies to intensify traditional control efforts. For example, Harris County worked with Project Premonition to test robotic traps for mosquitoes that can remotely determine the species by wing movement. Lee County, Florida, is using drones to control nuisance mosquitoes in hard to reach mangrove areas.

Nearby, 20,000 male mosquitoes infected with a naturally occurring bacteria, *Wolbachia*, were released in the Florida Keys in 2017–an area that experienced a dengue outbreak in 2009. When males infected with *Wolbachia* mate with female mosquitoes, the bacteria affect the eggs so that they will not hatch, resulting in a reduced or eliminated mosquito population.

While these new technologies hold significant promise, communities must be engaged *before* investments are made to determine if there is public support. Drones flying over neighborhoods, releases of *Wolbachia*-infected or genetically modified mosquitoes, all have the potential to draw concern from residents. Experts and public health officials are quickly learning that the biggest roadblock to introducing new control measures can be rooted within the very communities they are intended to help.

This became evident when the Florida Keys Mosquito Control District wanted to introduce genetically modified male mosquitoes after that 2009 outbreak. Despite a near-decade-long process of obtaining government approvals and engaging the community through town halls, referendums, and educational sessions no release has been conducted, in large part due to community opposition.

Many people were–and still are–opposed to anything that is genetically modified, even though the result would be the same as the *Wolbachia* bacteria–infected mosquitos: reducing the population through sterilization.

Preventive Measures

As with most advances, some communities will have the resources to take advantage of these new technologies and some will not. The good news is that there are ways to mitigate risk of infection that anyone can take. Eliminating habitats for mosquitoes and ticks in private and public areas is critical. Any standing water is a hazard as it can create a breeding ground for mosquitoes. Public health officials recommend that *every week* residents empty and scrub, turn over, cover, or throw out items that hold water–such as tires, buckets, planters, toys, pools, birdbaths, flowerpots or trash containers.

Many people may not realize that some mosquitoes–like the one that transmits Zika–can even lay eggs in containers inside the home, so it is important to check flower vases and containers. And, of course, contact with mosquitoes can be reduced by wearing repellent or longer clothing and screening doors and windows.

Unfortunately, not all people have the resources to adhere to these standard public health recommendations. Making home repairs and purchasing repellent on a regular basis may be out of reach for some of the most vulnerable populations. Therefore, identifying key barriers to the implementation of prevention tactics is a critical gap in current public health recommendations.

Engaging the whole community is critical. After all, it's entirely possible that while you are on top of these recommended chores, your neighbor may not be. In past surveys we have conducted in Key West and Tucson, we've noted that of the people who reported a reason for not being able to remove standing water, one in 10 indicated they were physically unable to do so. Assisting neighbors in removing or treating standing water will aid in the protection and health of the entire community.

It's crucial that public officials open a conversation with community members to ensure they are knowledge partners every step of the way, to provide a forum for discussion and to assuage concerns about the newest technologies, to ensure communities know what is necessary to make sure mosquitoes aren't welcome, and to assist the community members who need help with upkeep in their own yards. Organizing entire communities to understand the risk—and then react to it—is the only way to start to address this increasing threat to health.

The views expressed are those of the author(s) and are not necessarily those of Scientific American.

About the Author

Kacey C. Ernst, PhD, MPH, is an associate professor and program director of epidemiology at the University of Arizona's Mel and Enid Zuckerman College of Public Health and a 2017 AAAS Leshner Fellow for Public Engagement. Her primary projects examine the environmental determinants of vector-borne disease transmission and control. She and a team recently developed the Kidenga app.

Want to Prevent Another Coronavirus Epidemic?

By William A. Haseltine

Once again we stand unprepared as the third epidemic of a new and deadly coronavirus races around the world. This need not have been the case.

We should have learned from the SARS epidemic of 2003, which claimed nearly 800 lives, that coronaviruses can turn deadly. Until then, most health officials and scientists regarded coronaviruses simply as one of many causes of the common cold; some 30 percent of common colds start from coronaviruses. Then came the MERS epidemic in the Middle East in 2012, a coronavirus that killed 858 people. The irrefutable lesson from SARS and MERS: coronaviruses can spread quickly and be deadly.

Why, then, is there no way to prevent or treat the disease in 2020? Science had the tools in the immediate aftermath of the previous two epidemics to develop the drugs to control future outbreaks. But health officials, scientists and governments, especially but not only in the United States and China, dropped the ball.

There is no doubt that coronaviruses are wily opponents. Like all viruses of this type, the coronavirus mixes and matches components to create novel versions of itself. Bats are the natural hosts of the virus. There are more than 1,100 species of bats, each infected with one or more coronavirus variants. Think of the virus as a genetic safecracker, constantly evolving new combinations to extend its range and find new host species. Humans are on that menu. Each infection, deadly or not, is different from the last, which makes an effective vaccine or cure for the whole family of coronaviruses highly unlikely.

Though we may not be able to develop a cure for those already ill, we can develop drugs that will prevent the disease from spreading. If we had done so after SARS and MERS, governments could have stockpiled the drugs years in advance of this latest outbreak and within one-day delivery to all locations where the virus has been detected or suspected. All patients, hospital workers and any other persons suspected of contact would have been treated to stop the epidemic in its tracks.

I led the effort to develop an effective drug to prevent and treat anthrax following the 2001 attack and was a pioneer for the concept of using drugs to prevent transmission of HIV/AIDS from mother to child and between adults. Assessing the genome of this new virus, I see what we describe as a "target-rich" environment; that is, a virus that has many vulnerabilities to antiviral drugs, similar to those that have been exploited successfully for the treatment of HIV, hepatitis B and herpes viruses. The drugs, or combinations of drugs, that control those diseases bind and block the enzymes the viruses need to grow.

These enzymes are very similar to one another in all coronaviruses. This is a critical point. This common molecular pattern of all coronaviruses makes the challenge of identifying drugs to control coronaviruses less daunting. Scientists design drugs to inhibit the growth of specific virus enzymes. Once the genetic code of a virus has been sequenced, the targets for effective drugs appear.

We now have witnessed three deadly coronavirus outbreaks in humans within 17 years. Once this new epidemic has faded into memory, will it be five or 10 years until the next one? We can and must develop, test and stockpile combinations of drugs that can protect against what is certain to be another coronavirus outbreak.

In the wake of the 9/11 attacks, the U.S. government established the legal authority and executive process to do this. Known as BioShield, the program authorized funding to develop and stockpile effective means to prevent and treat "new and emerging biological threats." BioShield works. At Human Genome Sciences we developed the drug Abthrax to prevent and cure anthrax infections after the 2001 attacks. That drug is now stockpiled by the government. BioShield created the market for our work, committing many millions of dollars in purchase orders.

The coronavirus is not now and has never been on BioShield's approved list of "new and emerging biological threats." It should have been added after SARS, then again after MERS. It should be added now. We have been forewarned.

The departments of Homeland Security, Health and Human Services, and Defense should convene a working group immediately to add coronaviruses to the BioShield agenda. The Centers for Disease Control and National Institutes of Health then can initiate contractual discussions with the biopharmaceutical industry. Biopharmaceutical companies have the expertise to create the drugs we need quickly to prevent a fourth outbreak.

Collectively, scientists at these agencies and companies then can, and will, soon identify the drugs and produce the stockpiles that we need, that the world needs, to prevent a fourth deadly outbreak from a coronavirus, any coronavirus.

The views expressed are those of the author(s) and are not necessarily those of Scientific American.

About the Author

William A. Haseltine is a former Harvard Medical School professor and founder of the university's cancer and HIV/AIDS research departments. He also serves as chair and president of the global health think tank ACCESS Health International. He has founded more than a dozen biotechnology companies and is the author, most recently, of Variants! The Shape-Shifting Challenge of COVID-19.

The Next Zika

By Marta Zaraska

Disease detectives are on the lookout for obscure viruses that can be spread among people by traveling insects, and quickly become a widespread problem. Scientific papers are filled with illnesses to watch. Four particular viruses now stand out to virologists and epidemiologists, although it is not certain any of the ailments will become the next Zika or West Nile virus. But researchers give several reasons to keep a close eye on this quartet:

Mayaro

"For 10 years now I've been thinking that Mayaro is right on the cusp of being able to amplify in humans and being transmitted efficiently by *Aedes aegypti* mosquitoes," says Scott Weaver, a virologist at The University of Texas Medical Branch at Galveston. Mayaro causes a disease that is clinically indistinguishable from the mosquito-borne chikungunya virus: fever, chills, rash and the characteristic joint pain that can last longer than a year. It does matter, though, which of these viruses circulates in your body. Once there are vaccines against Mayaro and chikungunya, and drugs to treat them (so far there are none), they will likely be virus-specific.

Similarities with chikungunya are also why Mayaro might become a widespread problem. Both were originally transmitted by forest mosquitoes, infecting people in places like the Amazonia. Yet chikungunya has already adapted to be transmitted by urban mosquitoes, such as *A. aegypti* or *Aedes albopictus*–as of September 2016 in the Americas alone there were over 100,000 confirmed cases of the disease. Such adaptations may be happening with Mayaro, too. In lab experiments *A. aegypti* and *A. albopictus* have been shown as potential vectors for Mayaro. What's more, in recent years there were cases in large Brazilian cities–far from forests. In September 2016 the virus was detected in Haiti, further suggesting possible adaptations to an urban cycle. "It could just be that the right strain was introduced into that area or it could be that the virus has mutated to facilitate urban transmission," Weaver says.

Rift Valley Fever

For most people, a Rift Valley infection means a simple illness of fever and chills. Yet in some it can progress to a hemorrhagic disease, accompanied by abnormal bleeding, or to inflammation of the brain. Half of Rift Valley hemorrhagic cases are fatal, and there is no treatment.

Since its discovery in Kenya in the early 20th century, the Rift Valley virus has been limited to Africa. But in 2000 it left the continent, reaching the Arabian Peninsula. By 2014 there have been numerous outbreaks causing tens of thousands of human cases and millions of livestock deaths. In recent years more people have ended up with the hemorrhagic disease (10 percent versus 1 percent from early observations). "The jury is still out whether the virus is mutating to be more virulent or, more likely, we are just much better at detecting severe infections in Africa," says Brian Bird, a virologist at the University of California, Davis School of Veterinary Medicine One Health Institute.

The problem with Rift Valley fever is that it can be spread by over 30 species of mosquitoes, 19 of them native to North America. Both wild and domestic animals can serve as a reservoir of the disease. "The availability of immunologically naive livestock to perpetuate the disease in North America or in Europe is concerning. If it were to come here, the effects on animal health and economy would be profound," Bird says. A likely way for Rift Valley fever to arrive into the U.S. would be via virus-carrying mosquitoes on airplanes or ships. Luckily, the work on a vaccine is quite advanced.

Crimean–Congo Hemorrhagic Fever

Crimean–Congo hemorrhagic fever is transmitted by ticks—which is good news because tick-borne infections are likely to spread more slowly than mosquito-carried ones. The bad news is that Crimean–Congo has fatality rates up to 40 percent. Identified in 1944, the virus has already managed to travel from Africa all the way to China. In recent years the virus's spread seems to have accelerated: In 2002 it arrived in Turkey, infecting 10,000 people by 2015; by 2011 the virus reached India; and in September 2016 the first two cases were registered in Spain. One person died. "It's very difficult to say if that was a one-off introduction of the virus or an indicator of changes in the environment allowing the virus to spread to this area of Europe," Bird says.

Besides bleeding from almost anywhere in the body, the disease can cause rash and fever. The antiviral drug ribavirin has been used to treat Crimean–Congo, but it is not very effective.

The virus is transmitted by ticks, mostly from the *Hyalomma* genus, that with climate change are creeping into new territories. They have already been found as far north as Germany (in 2015) and even in the U.K., hitchhiking on migratory birds. Whether there are ticks that could transmit Crimean–Congo in North America remains unknown.

Usutu

"After an unusually warm summer in Europe we are facing an unprecedented outbreak of Usutu among birds in Germany, a massive die-off, and colleagues from France, Belgium, Hungary, the Netherlands are also reporting similar phenomena. That's new—earlier Usutu outbreaks were always limited geographically," says Daniel Cadar, virologist at Bernhard–Nocht Institute for Tropical Medicine in Hamburg.

Usutu, an avian virus transmitted by commonplace *Culex* mosquitoes, causes a disease that is a West Nile virus fever lookalike: headaches, fever, neurological problems. But so far, most Usutu infections in humans end without symptoms. According to a study published this September in *Clinical Microbiology and Infection*, over 6 percent of Italians around Modena have been recently and unknowingly infected with the virus. Serious symptoms are most likely to occur in people with compromised immunity, as it was reported in 2013 in Croatia–on just three cases. Yet Weaver says we shouldn't underestimate this infection. "Usutu is not far from where West Nile fever was 20 years ago. There were some small outbreaks in eastern Europe, but for the most part people thought it was not a serious pathogen. Because Usutu is an avian virus, it could easily circulate in many different parts of the world, just like West Nile virus," he cautions. And climate change could mean more infected birds, and more potential for human–virus contact, too.

About the Author

Marta Zaraska, a freelance writer based in France, is author of Growing Young: How Friendship, Optimism and Kindness Can Help You Live to 100 *(Penguin Random House, 2020). She wrote "Shrinking Animals" in the June 2018 issue of* Scientific American.

COVID Is Here to Stay

By Christine Crudo Blackburn

COVID-19 will continue in pandemic form, surging in one or more regions and disrupting daily life, until the world reaches herd immunity. With that, most scientists say, the SARS-CoV-2 virus will become endemic—always present but transmitted among people at modest, predictable rates. After several years the infamous 1918 influenza pandemic made that transition, and the virus is still circulating, 104 years later, in mutated strains. Almost all influenza A infections since 1918 have descended from that strain.

As the endemic stage arrives, people of all ages will be eligible for the COVID vaccine, and hospitals and pharmacies will be well supplied with effective treatments for infection. At that point, it might be wise for public health officials to treat COVID as a respiratory disease that is more dangerous than a cold, similar to how we handle influenza and cytomegalovirus (CMV)—by evaluating distribution of a seasonal vaccine, tracking hospitalization rates and educating the public about current risk. We don't yet know if COVID will lead to higher rates of long-term complications than those diseases do, so other precautions may be necessary.

In this future, routine testing might become part of everyday life. People with imperceptible symptoms who test positive would know to wear masks and isolate from others. If we could develop similar tests for influenza and CMV and make them cheaply available to everyone, everywhere, society could end up even safer against infectious respiratory diseases than it was before COVID arrived.

Even if COVID cases declined significantly, it's unlikely the virus would burn out. As long as it was still spreading in animals, it could spill over into humans at another time. Nature is always surprising us. A future, reemergent SARS-CoV-2 could be either less or more transmissible, less or more lethal. The Omicron variant that spread this winter taught us to expect the unexpected. Our world still has much to do to become better prepared for new variants—as well as whatever novel virus emerges next.

About the Author

Christine Crudo Blackburn is an assistant professor of security studies at Sam Houston State University.

GLOSSARY

antibiotic A substance that kills microorganisms.

epidemic A disease with a sudden and widespread outbreak.

epidemiology A branch of medical science that deals with disease in a population.

inflammatory Having to do with a bodily response to injury or disease in which part of the body becomes warm, red, and swollen.

inoculation Vaccination that introduces portions of a pathogen into the body to stimulate antibodies.

pandemic A disease that spreads very quickly throughout the whole world.

pathogen A microorganism (such as a bacterium or virus) that causes a specific disease.

polarization Division into extreme opposites, especially beliefs or interests.

quarantine Keeping something away from the public to stop the spread of disease.

vector A creature that spreads disease from one source to another.

zoonotic A disease that can be transferred from one animal to another, usually to humans.

FURTHER INFORMATION

Anthes, Emily. "Could the Next Pandemic Start at the County Fair?," *New York Times*, July 25, 2023, https://www.nytimes.com/2023/07/25/health/swine-flu-pigs-agriculture.html.

Archibong, Belinda, Francis Annan, and Uche Ekhator-Mobayode. "The Epidemic Effect: Epidemics, Institutions, and Human Capital Investment," Brookings Institution, June 14, 2023, https://www.brookings.edu/articles/the-epidemic-effect-epidemics-institutions-and-human-capital-development/.

"Epidemic and Pandemic-Prone Diseases," World Health Organization, https://www.emro.who.int/pandemic-epidemic-diseases/outbreaks/index.html.

"Epidemic, Endemic, Pandemic: What are the Differences?," Columbia Mailman School of Public Health, February 19, 2021, https://www.publichealth.columbia.edu/news/epidemic-endemic-pandemic-what-are-differences.

Robinson, Dana, and Ann Battenfield. "The Worst Outbreaks in U.S. History," Healthline, May 10, 2023, https://www.healthline.com/health/worst-disease-outbreaks-history.

Uddin, Nizam, and Thamina Acter. "An Overview of Global Epidemics and the Challenges Faced," *Leveraging Artificial Intelligence in Global Epidemics*, August 6, 2021, https://www.ncbi.nlm.nih.gov/pmc/articles/PMC8342595/.

Weintraub, Karen. "The Next Pandemic Could Spring from U.S. Meat Supply, New Report Finds," *USA Today*, July 23, 2023, https://www.usatoday.com/story/news/health/2023/07/22/deadly-covid-style-pandemic-could-easily-start-in-us-report-finds/70442786007/.

CITATIONS

1.1 100 Years after the Lethal 1918 Flu Pandemic, We Are Still Vulnerable by Catharine I. Paules and Anthony S. Fauci (September 15, 2017); 1.2 The 1918 Flu Faded in Our Collective Memory: We Might 'Forget' the Coronavirus, Too by Scott Hershberger (August 13, 2020); 1.3 Lessons from Past Outbreaks Could Help Fight the Coronavirus Pandemic by Sara Goudarzi (March 23, 2020); 1.4 Stories from a Past Pandemic by The Editors (January 28, 2021); 1.5 Millions of People Living with HIV Are Alive, Thanks to a 20-Year Public Health Effort by Lauren J. Young (March 27, 2023); 1.6 HIV Care Has Improved Dramatically–But Not for Everyone by David Malebranche (June 1, 2022); 1.7 Lessons from AIDS for the COVID-19 Pandemic by William A. Haseltine (October 1, 2020); 2.1 How China's 'Bat Woman' Hunted Down Viruses from SARS to the New Coronavirus by Jane Qiu (June 1, 2020); 2.2 A High-Speed Scientific Hive Mind Emerged from the COVID Pandemic by Joseph Bak-Coleman and Carl T. Bergstrom (March 1, 2022); 2.3 An mRNA Pioneer Discusses How Her Work Led to the COVID Vaccines by Tanya Lewis (September 15, 2021); 2.4 Messenger RNA Therapies Are Finally Fulfilling Their Promise by Drew Weissman (March 1, 2022); 2.5 Pandemic-Era Research Will Pay Off for Years by Britt Glaunsinger (March 1, 2022); 2.6 COVID Revealed the Fragility of American Public Health by Wendy E. Parmeton (March 1, 2022); 2.7 COVID Pushed Global Health Institutions to Their Limits by Lawrence O. Gostin (March 1, 2022); 3.1 COVID Has Made Global Inequality Much Worse by Joseph E. Stiglitz (March 1, 2022); 3.2 COVID Has Created a Perfect Storm for Fringe Science by David Robert Grimes (April 26, 2021); 3.3 COVID Changed the World of Work Forever by Christina Maslach and Michael P. Leiter (March 1, 2022); 3.4 How a Virus Exposed the Myth of Rugged Individualism by Robin G. Nelson (March 1, 2022); 3.5 How the Pandemic Remade Science Journalism by Tanya Lewis (March 1, 2022); 3.6 Introducing 21 Ways COVID Changed the World by Jen Schwartz (March 1, 2022); 4.1 The Biggest Health Problem: Obesity by Mercedes Carnethon (June 21, 2019); 4.2 The Opioid Epidemic Is Surging among Black People because of Unequal Access to Treatment by Melba Newsome and Gioncarlo Valentine (December 1, 2022); 4.3 Doctors Need to Learn to Talk about Suicide by Rodolfo Bonnin and Leonard M. Gralnik (August 26, 2022); 4.4 Why Does Ebola Keep Showing Up in the Democratic Republic of the Congo? by Dina Fine Maron (May 11, 2018); 4.5 Ebola Outbreak in Uganda Surges, but the Country Has a Plan by Paul Adepoju (October 13, 2022); 4.6 'Their Lives Are Worth More Than Ours': Experts in Africa Slam Global Response to Monkeypox by Paul Adepoju (July 27, 2022); 4.7 We Can't Let Monkeypox Turn into a Repeat of COVID by Muhammad Jawad Noon (June 23, 2022); 5.1 Tick- and Mosquito-Borne Diseases Are Increasing Dramatically by Kacey C. Ernst (August 10, 2018); 5.2 Want to Prevent Another Coronavirus Epidemic? by William A. Haseltine (January 29, 2020); 5.3 The Next Zika by Marta Zaraska (October 11, 2016); 5.4 COVID Is Here to Stay by Christine Crudo Blackburn (March 1, 2022).

Each author biography was accurate at the time the article was originally published.

INDEX

A

animal origins of diseases, 8, 10, 17, 53–62, 80–81, 122–124, 129, 141–145, 146, 149–152
antigenic drift, 9, 10
antiretrovirals, 30, 33, 37, 41, 45
antivirals, 8, 49, 75, 147, 151

B

bacterial infections, 8, 71

C

Centers for Disease Control and Prevention (CDC), 19, 30, 82, 99, 113, 118, 123, 148
climate change and disease, 78, 141–142, 151, 152
Crimean-Congo hemorrhagic fever, 151
coronaviruses, 19, 43, 47–48, 53, 55–58, 78
  preventing another epidemic, 146–148
COVID-19, 13, 14, 27, 128, 130, 133, 135, 136–139
  American public health and, 76–77
  American "rugged individualism" and, 94–97
  becoming endemic, 153–154
  collective memory and, 12–18
  containment procedures, 13, 15, 20–21, 47, 65, 79, 82, 90, 95, 99–100, 137–138, 153
  deaths from, 19, 48, 53–54, 102, 138
  early days of, 53, 57, 58–62, 63–65
  inequality and, 85–87, 103, 110, 138
  journalism/media coverage of, 16, 63, 98–101, 102
  misinformation/disinformation about, 65, 88–91, 98, 99–100, 102–103, 136, 138
  origin of, 58–60, 80–81
  research on, 47–49, 63–66, 75
  treatment for, 46, 49
  using lessons from the past to fight, 19–23, 41–51
  vaccine, 15, 43–44, 61, 64, 67–71, 72–74, 75, 81, 82, 86–87, 88, 95, 96,

99–100, 102, 104, 133, 136, 138, 153
work life and, 92–93

E

Ebola, 19, 36, 78
in Democratic Republic of the Congo, 122–125
in Uganda, 126–130

F

Fauci, Dr. Anthony, 6, 8–11, 49
"forgetting" of pandemics, 12–18, 24, 25

G

global health institutions and COVID, 78–82

H

HIV/AIDS
barriers to treatment, 37–40
funding for research, 47–49
prevention, 33–34, 38, 40, 46–47, 147
statistics on, 41, 46
treatment for, 30–36, 37–40, 41–42, 44–46
vaccine for, 42–44, 73

I

immunity, 9, 10–11, 22–23, 43, 153
inequality and epidemics/pandemics, 85–87, 103, 106–108, 109–117, 133–134, 138, 144
influenza, 19–20, 153
deaths from, 8, 9, 12, 19, 24
pandemic of 1918, 8–11, 12–13, 14–18, 19, 20–21, 24–29, 153
seasonal epidemics, 9–10, 22–23
vaccine for 8, 9–11, 73

M

masks, and disease prevention, 13, 27, 65, 79, 82, 90, 95, 99–100, 137, 153
MERS, 47, 48, 146, 148
monkeypox, 36, 131–135, 136–139
mosquito-borne diseases, 141–145, 149, 150, 151

N

National Institutes of Health, 10, 44, 111, 116

O

obesity, epidemic of, 106–108
opioid epidemic, 109–117

P

political polarization/divides, 15, 41, 99–100, 102–103, 138
pseudoscience, 88–91

Q

quarantine/isolation, 20, 21, 50, 82, 85, 94–95, 153

R

Rift Valley virus, 150

S

SARS, 19, 21, 22, 47–48, 53, 55–57, 60, 146, 148
Shi Zhengli ("bat woman"), 53–62
social distancing, 13, 15, 20–21, 65, 95
suicide, 118–121
swine flu, 17, 19

T

tick-borne diseases, 141–145, 151

U

Usutu, 151–152

V

vaccines, 8, 41, 42, 149, 150
- anti-vaxxers, 89, 99, 100
- COVID-19, 15, 43–44, 61, 64, 67–71, 72–74, 75, 81, 82, 86–87, 88, 95, 96, 99–100, 102, 104, 133, 136, 138, 153
- Ebola, 126, 130
- influenza, 8, 9–11, 73
- monkeypox/smallpox, 132, 133–134, 138
- mRNA, 64, 67–71, 72–74, 75, 81–82, 100, 102

W

West Nile virus, 142, 149, 151–152
World Health Organization (WHO), 19, 30, 64, 78, 88, 90, 99, 124, 131, 132, 135, 136–138

Z

Zika, 19, 73, 78, 143, 144, 149